The Cesarean Birth Experience

A Practical, Comprehensive and
Reassuring Guide for Parents
and Professionals

Completely Revised and Updated

Bonnie Donovan

Beacon Press
Boston

Beacon Press
25 Beacon Street
Boston, Massachusetts 02108

Beacon Press books are published under the auspices
of the Unitarian Universalist Association
of Congregations in North America.

First edition published 1977. Revised edition 1986.

Printed in the United States of America

92 91 90 89 88 87 86   8 7 6 5 4 3 2 1

Library of Congress Cataloging in Publication Data

Donovan, Bonnie.
    The cesarean birth experience.

    Bibliography: p.
    Includes index.
    1. Cesarean section.   I. Title.   [DNLM: 1. Cesarean
Section—popular works. WQ 150 D687c]
RG761.D66   1985   618.8′6   85–47520
ISBN 0–8070–2701–4

I lovingly dedicate this book to Jon and Sarah, who caused this book to be written; to my husband, Steven Koepple; to my mother, Evon Krusher; to my father, Frederick Rose; to my aunts and uncles, especially Marion, Madeline, and Loree; to my dear friend Beverly Trainer; and to Carol S. and William A. Donovan.

And forever, to R.M.A.

CONTENTS

Acknowledgments   ix

How It All Began   xi

Foreword   xv

1   The Cesarean Difference   1

2   Indications: Why Me?   7

3   Pregnancy   38

4   Emotional Stress: The Fear Factor   59

5   Tests to Determine Fetal Maturity
and Well-being   77

6   Signs of Labor and What to Do   93

7   Preparing for the Birth: Hospital Admissions
and Routines   97

8   Birthday!   114

9   The Recovery Room: A Good Beginning   133

10   The Postpartum Hospital Stay   143

11   The "Fourth" Trimester   160

12   Human Bonding: The Importance of Touching
and the Advantages of Breast-feeding   177

13   History and Evolution
            of the Cesarean Delivery   195

14   Choices to Explore: A Checklist   203

15   Education and Support   207

16   Subsequent Vaginal Delivery:
            The VBAC Option   223

            Conclusion: The Way It Should Be   246

            Resources/Organizations   248

            Notes   250

            Suggested Reading   254

            Index   257

ACKNOWLEDGMENTS

My husband, Steven, and my children, Jon and Sarah, cannot be thanked enough for all that they have endured and sacrificed in the nine months it required to update this book.

Special appreciation to Esther Booth Zorn and Nancy Edwards Dow, M.D., who were gracious and generous. Of course I am and always will be particularly indebted to Ruth M. Allen, R.N., M.S., British-trained nurse-midwife, childbirth educator, lecturer, and pathfinder.

Thanks also to Muriel Sugarman, M.D., Elisabeth Bing, R.P.T., Valmai Elkins, R.P.T., Elizabeth Caswell, R.N., and John Caswell, R.N., Leslie and Fred Hill, Linda Peterson, Maeva Buckman, R.N., Ruth Rotko, and Neil Weisbrod, and the staff of South Shore Hospital, South Weymouth, Massachusetts.

And of course, thank you Mischa Askren, M.D., and Stephanie for helping light the way.

Deepest thanks to Joanne Wyckoff who bore up nobly with transcontinental editing. Also, I must extend a word of gratitude to Gregg-Edward Moscoe, my friend and sometime agent.

HOW IT ALL BEGAN

When this book was first published in 1977, it was the culmination of years of work, research, and study. It was also the result of some very supportive cesarean parents and empathetic professionals. I did not, initially, intend to write a book. All I wanted was to make sure that my second cesarean was better, less devastating, less traumatic, than my first one. I searched and searched for answers and found none.

Being tenacious, I started digging deeper and deeper into the subject. My efforts seemed futile and discouraging. Was I the only cesarean mother who was grateful to have had a healthy baby but confused and overwhelmed by the emotional aftermath and total lack of information? Were my husband and I the only ones who wanted prepared cesarean childbirth education and books to read? Were we the only parents who wanted to share the cesarean birth of our baby together? Was I the only woman who went to two states and a dozen different obstetricians, trying to find one who would let me go into labor spontaneously, rather than insist that I submit to a scheduled repeat cesarean? Were there other parents who thirsted for information and empathy? Were there any doctors, nurses, midwives, or childbirth educators who would listen to my requests for education and family-centered cesarean birth? The answers to the last two questions were a resounding, "Yes!" Unsolicited, five thousand orders came flooding in for copies of the book I had not yet even finished writing. And when I searched for supportive doctors, nurses, midwives, and childbirth educators, slowly but surely a few open-minded professionals came to my aid.

What began as a strictly personal quest for information on a subject which was, at the time, totally shrouded in medical mystery and thoroughly obscured from the parental perspective, resulted in a book that helped thousands of other cesarean parents demystify and illuminate the subject of cesarean childbirth. Like you, I was just an average parent-to-be. I could never have written this book alone. Parents called me and wrote long letters. They opened their hearts to offer encouragement for the project and shared with me their experiences, their expectations, their suggestions. A few brave doctors and nurses (Ruth Allen, most particularly) took me under their wings and patiently taught me medical terms and practices. They explained procedures and philosophies. They allowed me to attend lectures and seminars open only to professionals within the fields of obstetrics and childbirth education. They offered me their erudite opinions, corrected technical errors, and, sometimes at great risk or inconvenience to themselves, cut through red tape so that I could go on rounds with them and attend (with the parents' permission, of course) many cesarean and vaginal hospital births. Thanks to caring, open-minded midwives, I was able to drive through the snows of Vermont and the redwood forests of California to watch with wonder and delight as home births took place.

Oddly enough, revising this book was no less easy than writing it from scratch. In one respect, it was even more difficult. That is because I wanted you to know that you are not alone, that someone (in fact, many people) care about you and want to help you achieve the best possible birth experience. This time, I have included more information on why many routine interventions into pregnancy, labor and delivery should be shunned or at least carefully considered rather than automatically accepted. I have provided information on how you may be able to *prevent* a first-time or repeat cesarean. I have also supplied information on subsequent vaginal delivery. Vaginal birth after cesarean (or other uterine surgery) is now commonly known as VBAC. VBAC does not have to be a dream; more often than not it is possible to achieve. Abolishing all but a small percentage of cesareans is clearly imperative. What I do not want, however, is for you to feel like a failure if you end up having a cesarean—either because it is medically mandated or because you cannot, in time for your birth, find appropriate resources within your community to support you in this endeavor. It is time to fight fire with fire. You have a responsibility to yourself and your baby to know that many—in fact, most—cesareans are unnecessary. Even obstetricians admit that this is so. Unless dramatic steps are taken immediately, you may have a cesarean section for a vague, avoidable, ambiguous, or even wrong reason. Be assured that cesarean delivery is safer than most operations; but it is still an operation and one to which you should not submit unless it is imperative in order to protect you or your baby from high risk or certain death.

It is no longer enough to know that cesarean parents have available to them all the components that contribute to a warm, joyful, comfortable, family-centered cesarean birth. Do not be lulled into thinking that all cesareans are acceptable today because of family-centered cesarean care. This simply is not so. However, if you have already given birth by cesarean, for whatever reason, the fact is that you cannot change what has already happened. You are a cesarean parent and you are in need of information that will explain what happened to you and why. What's more, you will need reassurance and encouragement to help you have positive feelings about yourself and the method of your baby's birth.

In our righteous zeal to abolish all but a small percentage of cesareans, we cannot and should not overlook two critical factors: (1) As unfortunate as it is, the incidence of cesareans will not plummet as fast as it skyrocketed; and (2) Even when the incidence is lowered to 5 percent or any fraction of what it is now, there will always be a certain number of parents who must give birth by cesarean. Cesarean parents will continue to need support, information, education, and understanding. In our stampede to eradicate all but a very, very few justifiable cesareans, we must not trample over the remaining parents who must have their babies in this manner.

Bonnie Donovan-Koepple
January 1986
Los Angeles, California

FOREWORD

It has been almost a decade since Bonnie Donovan first gave this book to women. *The Cesarean Birth Experience* was the first book to focus on cesarean birth and to explain how parents-to-be could prepare for and cope with the experience. *The Cesarean Birth Experience* of 1986 still provides this very necessary information and support, but it has grown with the times and now provides much more.

Most of you who pick up *The Cesarean Birth Experience* will find the information you need to make informed choices. You will also find comforting answers to the many questions you have about your impending childbirth experience and about past ones as well. Women giving birth in the next two decades will be faced with increasingly more complicated issues surrounding childbirth. Technology and medical procedures are expanding, causing women to examine more closely their beliefs and value systems. I hope a variety of answers and choices will always be available.

The idea of Vaginal Birth After Cesarean (VBAC) and the concept of cesarean prevention are answers and choices that have emerged over the past ten years. When *The Cesarean Birth Experience* was first written nine years ago, my son was born by cesarean because of a failure-to-progress diagnosis. The U.S. cesarean rate at the time was about 17 percent. Since then I have birthed two children naturally, one in the hospital and one at home. The cesarean rate now is over 21 percent, and many hospitals report rates of 25 percent and higher. Therefore, it is now necessary to have the Cesarean Prevention Movement, an organization dedicated to lowering the cesarean rate.

Most of you who decide to read this book will not have to have a cesarean for medical reasons. In fact, after you read all that is entailed in having a cesarean you will most likely work harder to unload any physical, emotional, or psychological baggage that might keep you from experiencing birth as the normal physiological process that it is. Bringing a baby into this world by cesarean is very emotionally and physically taxing for everyone involved, especially the mother. With this book you will discover information about the cesarean procedure in detail and how you in most cases can remain an active participant. You will have an opportunity to learn the pros and cons of medical procedures and how to question their use. For those who must have a cesarean, Bonnie Donovan has provided a valuable resource. Those choosing a VBAC or wishing to prevent an unnecessary cesarean will find here very important information to start on a fascinating journey of discovery.

Esther Booth Zorn
Founding President
Cesarean Prevention Movement, Inc.

THE CESAREAN
BIRTH EXPERIENCE

THE CESAREAN DIFFERENCE

In terms of anatomy, the difference between a cesarean section and a vaginal delivery is a matter of a few inches. Yet the differences might just as well be measured in miles when we take into account the quality of the birth experience as seen from the parents' perspective, the additional risks of surgery, and the fact that many—if not most—cesareans are preventable.

As recently as 1968, there were only about 5 cesareans for every 100 births; today the figure is closer to 1 in 5. Until the past decade, the differences between a vaginal delivery and a cesarean section were not as great as they are today. Both types of births were routinely subjected to a multitude of medical interventions. For example, both vaginal delivery and cesarean mothers were routinely drugged during labor and "knocked out" with potent anesthesia for the birth. Only in the past decade or two have prepared childbirth classes become widely available and attended. The role of the father has been reassessed.

Today's climate of concern for pregnant couples is vastly improved. Both obstetricians and parents have become aware of the dangers of overmedicating birthing women or tampering too much with the normal course of labor and delivery.

Childbirth classes can now be found throughout the country and are offered by a variety of individuals and groups, each espousing some particular method—the Lamaze method, the Bradley method, the Leboyer method, and so on. And there are now many books that explore the joys, virtues, and controversies of prepared childbirth (see Suggested Reading). There are also general books on pregnancy, such as *Will My Baby Be Normal? How to Make Sure* by Jonathan Scher, M.D., and Carol Dix, as well as books that address themselves to cesarean birth, such as *How to Avoid a Cesarean Section* by Christopher Norwood. One of the newest additions to the bibliography of childbirth books is the timely *Silent Knife* by Nancy Wainer Cohen and Lois J. Estner, which straightforwardly criticizes the unpardonably high incidence of cesareans while at the same time offering comprehensive preventive measures (as does Norwood's book), and which addresses, for the first time in detail, the advantages of vaginal birth after cesarean (VBAC).

At last the essential role of the father (or a significant other) is almost universally recognized and encouraged. Although many men have been initially reluctant to attend childbirth classes, most soon become excited because they learn how important their support, encouragement, and presence are.

Family-Centered Maternity Care (FCMC) has now been implemented in all but the most outdated hospitals. The mother, father, and baby—as well as siblings, grandparents, and other close relatives—are now regarded as essential elements that contribute to the strength of the family. Some women give birth with both the father (or someone special) *and* a labor attendant (midwife, nurse, coach, advocate) present. Fathers and other family members are able to cuddle their newborns, rather than having to stare at them through the glass partitions of the hospital nursery. Alternative Birth Centers (ABCs), Normal Birth Centers (NBCs), rooming-in, and a host of other options are widely available. Breast-feeding continues to gain in popularity and cannot be encouraged enough.

Finding a comfortable, nonintrusive environment in which to have their babies has become a priority for many people. A number of parents are electing to give birth at home, for, despite ABCs, NBCs, and Family-Centered Maternity Care, these parents fear unwanted hospital intrusions or prefer the "risks" of staying home to the potential risks of medical interventions. It is interesting to note that Princess Diana of Great Britain initially wanted a home birth but was dissuaded from doing so. Nonetheless, she set a superb example for all modern mothers when she twice gave birth in an ABC and left the hospital within hours after the births of her sons. Perhaps this royal precedent gave other parents the courage to opt for nontraditional birthing places.

Cesarean parents, however, are still all too often the exceptions. They may still be the "odd" couple for whom everything is new, different, unexpected, and frightening. And their options are still often the most limited. Furthermore, with the emphasis on reducing the cesarean rate and encouraging more subsequent vaginal deliveries (even for women who've had more than one cesarean), it may now be all but impossible to approach childbirth without suspicion and the fear that you, too, will become a hapless victim of needless intervention and surgical delivery.

If this is your first cesarean, it is thoroughly understandable that you may have little knowledge about cesarean births. Most people envision the actual procedure only in terms of a doctor holding a knife poised over the mother's abdomen, blood gushing everywhere, and distraught fathers unable to do anything more than what all fathers used to do: pace about a waiting room somewhere agonizing over the fate of his mate and baby.

Although cesarean section is major surgery, it is still a

relatively safe operation. But just because it is safe does not mean that it is right to subject mothers and babies to the inherent risks of surgery *unless it is absolutely essential.*

THE GRAPEFRUIT SYNDROME

The cesarean mother, in her dual role as both postoperative *and* maternity patient, has special handicaps. In some hospitals she may be regarded as a nuisance because she needs more care and attention than her vaginally delivering counterpart. She may also be labeled "difficult" or "different" because she does not fit nicely into the category of motherhood as it is supposed to be. She is "the Section in room 204." No one has ever said, "There's a 'vag' down the hall." But there she is, "the Section in room 204." The section? It sounds as though we're talking about a grapefruit!

"Hah! You had your baby the easy way," friends tell the cesarean mother before they launch into tales of their own lengthy, difficult labors and deliveries. Her family may react differently: "Oh, you poor girl. You'll be crippled for life," they say as they wring their hands. Both attitudes are equally incorrect and damaging. There is certainly nothing easy about a cesarean delivery (be it an emergency after labor has begun or scheduled in advance of labor), nor does it mean that the mother will be an invalid as a result. The truth has been so clouded with myth and misinformation that cesarean parents may not know what to believe.

Most cesarean couples wish that they had been able to find out what happened to them and why. "What went wrong?" some ask. "What did I do that I shouldn't have?" "Why me?" "Why did this have to happen to me?" "What can I do to make the next time better?" Or, "How can I find out what happened, even though I know we'll never have another baby?"

As childbirth is seen in more "natural" terms, a great deal of emphasis is placed upon having one's baby with a maximum of understanding and preparation and a minimum of obstetrical management, drugs, and instrumentation. This is a very positive approach to childbirth. Because the traditional attitude regarding the cesarean delivery emphasizes the surgical rather than the birth aspect, cesarean mothers often feel left out and let down. It is dismaying to hear them refer to themselves as "failures" and natural childbirth "flunkies." This is not the way it has to be.

Fortunately, there is a growing awareness of the need to improve the cesarean birth experience. Individuals, childbirth education associations, and a growing number of doctors, nurses, and cesarean support groups have made greater advances in the past few years than at any time previously. Articles about the cesarean birth experience grace the pages of newspapers and magazines. Childbirth conferences now frequently include cesarean delivery as a topic of information and discussion. Classes have begun in many different locations for expectant cesarean couples. Cesarean prevention advocacy is just starting to stem the rising tide of unnecessary cesareans. These improvements are increasingly widespread, and pioneers in the field have seen what can be done when an effort is made to prepare cesarean parents through education and emotional support. In other words, the cesarean couple is now regarded in the same way as other parents and families and can be helped to have a positive, meaningful, fulfilling birth experience.

The term "cesarean section," in its numerous spellings and capitalizations, is the medical phrase for the procedure whereby a baby is delivered surgically instead of vaginally. I use the term when necessary for technical accuracy. However, when discussing the experience from an emotional and parental point of view, this book's primary objective, I feel that it is much more positive, much more reassuring, and much more to the point to use the words "cesarean birth" and "cesarean delivery," to emphasize the birth rather than the surgery. When we use the words "birth" and "delivery" in relation to the cesarean experience, it serves as a reminder that it is not just another surgical procedure—such as the removal of a tumor—but rather, and most important, the birth of a baby.

The Grapefruit Syndrome, like the "tension equals fear equals pain" philosophy, is cyclical. It is the cycle of fear, frustration, and stress that results from the almost total absence of practical information and reassuring support regarding cesarean birth. Although the physical needs of the cesarean mother and baby have been well met, until recently even the most well-intentioned health care professionals tended to neglect the emotional needs of the cesarean family.

The time is past for cesarean sections. It is now time for cesarean births and greater emphasis on cesarean prevention and subsequent vaginal deliveries.

INDICATIONS:
WHY ME?

Why me?!? is still the most frequent reaction to an emergency cesarean. Why did this have to happen to *me*? Was this fate, or was it my fault? Could this have been one of those avoidable cesareans?

Parents usually are willing to accept their doctors' explanations for what (allegedly) went wrong and why such drastic intervention was necessary. Even so, mothers tend to feel guilty, blaming themselves for something they think they did wrong or for having a "bad" attitude which contributed, at least in their minds, to the need for a cesarean.

The bottom line is this: Indications (that is, medical reasons) for cesarean delivery are often vague, ambiguous (even to the point of being arbitrary within the medical profession itself), and may have been performed on mothers and babies who were not even clearly at risk.

Regardless of the reason for the cesarean, and whether or not it was mandatory and unavoidable, here are some of the emotions expressed by cesarean parents:

"I couldn't believe that it could happen to me. Not to me. We had everything so nicely planned. My husband came to

classes and really wanted to help me through labor. But especially we wanted to share the birth of our baby. We wanted to see her arrival together."

"Cesareans happen to other *women. I did everything right [good prenatal care, proper diet and exercise, reading, attending classes, etc.]. Why did I end up with a section?"*

"I hated my baby for being too big to come out normally. I despised myself for taking the medication during labor. If only I hadn't done that, maybe I could have avoided having a c-section."

"If only the doctor had let me push longer."

"The nurse was such a witch. She made me get uptight. That's why I had a cesarean. I couldn't stay in touch with my body with her bugging me all the time."

"For some reason I felt that my husband was to blame for all this. I know he wasn't—I really wanted a baby—but I just got so angry with him for putting me through this terrible thing."

"My mother had two sections. She said she almost died both times. More than anything in the world, I wanted to avoid this."

"When the doctor told my husband to leave, because they were going to do a section, I felt both terrified and relieved. I hated having my husband go—he really helped a lot. But another part of me said, 'Thank God. Thank God. At last it's going to be all over. I won't feel this pain any more.'"

"All my friends have had babies naturally. One of them even delivered at home. She said it was the most beautiful time of her life. The others all had their husbands there for labor and delivery. I was too chicken to even think about having a baby at home. But we sure looked forward to having Bob there. He had his camera all ready. We talked for hours at a time about what it would be like to see our baby born. Sure, I wanted my baby to be healthy, but I could have killed the doctor when he made Bob leave me. I was so scared. I didn't think I could face it alone. I begged the doctor to put me out. I was afraid of the pain. I

didn't want to hear what was happening. Among all the other things I was thinking about, I kept flashing on the fact that I was going to be different. *I wouldn't be able to tell my friends about my baby's birth. I felt cheated. I was gypped. It wasn't my baby's fault, but I didn't like being left out."*

It used to be that when an expectant mother tried to find out why she had to have a cesarean, she was patted on the head and told by an avuncular, patronizing obstetrician, "Now, now, don't worry your pretty little head. Don't ask me to explain things you cannot possibly understand." Often parents were content with that answer. But now that people are more aware of themselves as health care consumers, they want to know why, what, and even how expensive the doctor's services will be. It is important for parents to know what the indications are for the cesarean. Knowing this will help them to deal more effectively and confidently with the situation. It may even help them to achieve a more positive birth experience or, at least, to view it from a better perspective.

An emergency cesarean is often a surprise, both to the couple *and* to the doctor. The expectant woman's pregnancy and early labor may have been perfectly normal; neither the doctor nor the couple saw the need for surgical delivery until just a few minutes, or perhaps a few hours, beforehand. There is usually no reason to suspect that vaginal delivery will not be possible until labor has progressed. The couple may have done everything within their control to ensure the healthy, uncomplicated delivery of their baby. The mother may have had good prenatal care, eaten the appropriate foods, taken her vitamins regularly, attended classes, practiced her relaxation-breathing techniques, exercised faithfully, gotten as much rest as she needed, and happily awaited the baby's birth. The father may have been just as supportive and helpful as possible. The couple may have read every book they could find on pregnancy and childbirth.

It is not unusual for the early stage of labor to progress in a manner that is unremarkable. Sometimes the doctor informs the couple in advance if the baby may have to be delivered by cesarean; for example, if the baby is in a breech position (see page 17).

"The doctor told me weeks in advance that the baby was breech and that if she didn't turn, I might have to have a cesarean. I kept hoping . . . wishing . . . willing her to turn. I completely blocked out the thought of a section and concentrated all my efforts on making her turn. I didn't want a section, but my wishful thinking didn't work."

Not all primary (first-time) cesareans are emergencies. There are some indications for performing a first-time cesarean that can be determined in advance. Some of these are diabetes, active herpes simplex, chronic illnesses, and pelvic insufficiency (the mother's pelvis is too small to accommodate the passage of a baby). These indications are rare.

But the point is that most often the decision to perform a primary emergency cesarean is not known until labor has advanced. The announcement may be devastating. It may, however, be greeted with relief as well as anguish. If the labor has been especially long, painful, or complicated, the doctor's decision carries the promise that at least something will happen and *soon.*

"Boy, was I glad! Labor was just awful. Within minutes after the doctor said he was going to take the baby, they gave me a spinal. Did that feel good! It was instant relief from all the pain. Now that I think about it, I'm not too keen on having to have another cesarean. But I sure didn't mind the first time . . . at least not till it was all over. Then I felt bad."

The couple who has been together for labor may suddenly be

separated for the cesarean. They should not be. One father, in the days when it was uncommon for the father to wait at the hospital for the birth, much less act as coach and supporter, told me that the doctor telephoned him to ask for his permission to make a little incision. Thinking the doctor meant an episiotomy, the father readily agreed. Hours later, upon arriving at his wife's side, the man was horrified to learn that the "little incision" was a cesarean section. As he said, "If anything had happened to them [his wife and baby], I would have killed myself for not being there."

Another father, told by the medical staff that he would have to wait in the lobby because they were going to "section the baby," thought they were going to cut the baby into pieces. He had heard an old wives' tale that babies were sometimes cut to pieces during difficult deliveries. We may laugh at this man's ignorance, but his experience serves as an example of why more information is necessary and why hospitals are sometimes remiss in their responsibility to act as a liaison between the doctor, mother-to-be, and expectant father.

Until the past few years, most fathers spent the hour or so it takes to perform a cesarean in waiting rooms and lobbies. They worried, fantasized, and agonized about what was happening to their wives. The mother, meanwhile, was the center of attention—none of it from the person she loved, trusted, and depended upon. One father who was made to wait in a corridor outside the delivery room described his experience as follows: "I was really freaked out. That thing [the intercom] kept paging people and in my panic I thought every call was for my wife and baby."

When an emergency cesarean is performed, it may be for one or a combination of reasons. Each case is based upon individual considerations and takes into account the mother's medical profile. The reasons for a friend's cesarean are not necessarily the same as for yours.

In the first two editions of *The Cesarean Birth Experience,* I divided cesarean indications into two categories: emergency and elective. These classifications are, of course, still applicable, but it now seems more appropriate to group indications into three types: mandatory, probable, and relative or possible. Bear in mind that there is some overlap and interchangability among these categories, and that there is a fair amount of controversy inherent in determining who will be able to avoid a cesarean and who will not.

MANDATORY INDICATIONS

Mandatory or absolute indications, in which cesarean delivery is clearly required in order to protect the mother and/or baby from death or great risk, are also the least frequently encountered. Some of the medical conditions which often require cesarean delivery are: complete placenta previa; hemorrhage; placenta abruptio; prolapsed umbilical cord; maternal pelvic contraction; and transverse lie.

Complete Placenta Previa. The placenta is the life support organ for the fetus. It is attached to the wall of the uterus; its function is to sustain and nourish the fetus during gestation. Placenta previa means that the placenta is partially or completely covering the opening of the cervix, thus endangering the baby's safe exit. Mild to severe bleeding during the second and third trimesters of pregnancy is a warning sign of this condition. This type of bleeding during pregnancy helps differentiate placenta previa from placenta abruptio (see below). If placenta previa is diagnosed, doctors prefer to give the fetus the benefits of as much maturation and growth in utero as is safe before performing a cesarean.

Hemorrhage. Severe maternal hemorrhage or bleeding during labor is also an "absolute" indication for cesarean delivery. Placenta previa and placenta abruptio are subcategories of this classification.

Placenta Abruptio. Normally the placenta (the

unborn baby's life-support system) remains attached to the wall of the uterus and is delivered after the baby. As the name implies, placenta abruptio is the abrupt, usually partial detachment of the placenta from the uterine wall. It may be cause for immediate cesarean delivery. There may be abdominal pain or vaginal bleeding. (Note: Any bleeding during pregnancy should be immediately reported to your health care provider).

Prolapsed Umbilical Cord. When the umbilical cord slips down before the presenting part of the baby, it is said to be prolapsed. (Presenting part of the baby means the part of the baby's body that would be delivered first vaginally; usually this is the baby's head, although a breech baby will present buttocks first or even feet first). When a cord prolapses during labor, it is pinched between the head or breech of the fetus and the pelvis with each contraction. To avoid further compression and to diminish the dangers of anoxia (lack of oxygen) to the baby, the doctor, nurse, or midwife will hold the baby up off the cord until a cesarean can be performed. A prolapsed cord can be determined during labor by vaginal examination or by a particular distress pattern on a fetal monitor. Thus, this is both an absolute indication and one that is usually determined on an emergency basis after labor has started.

Maternal Pelvic Contraction. In this instance, the medical use of the word contraction refers to an alteration in the size and/or shape of the woman's pelvis, not to the normal contractions which occur during labor. Of all the mandatory indications for cesarean delivery, this is the *least* common one, and certainly in this country and others where women are usually well nourished and otherwise healthy this indication is very rare. One exception is the woman who has a traumatic injury to the pelvis from a ski injury, car accident, etc. Otherwise, the pelvis is usually normal and adequate in size to permit passage of even a large baby.

Transverse Lie. When the fetus is in a position crosswise to the mother's body (i.e., with its head or feet neither up nor down but almost horizontal to the ground), this is called transverse lie. It is the most dangerous way for a baby to be positioned at the time of birth, for it means that vaginal delivery is impossible. Only a very tiny or dead baby can be delivered vaginally from this position. Anoxia is the major danger for a baby in this position who refuses to turn.

Transverse lie has always been an indication for cesarean delivery. Since this indication is usually known during pregnancy, you will have time to prepare for a cesarean birth. One way of making this a more normal birth—and avoiding the risk of scheduling a cesarean before the baby is fully mature—is to wait until you go into labor spontaneously.

PROBABLE INDICATIONS

Probable indications mean that there is some leeway regarding the method of delivery. Indications which fall into this category are: active genital herpes; eclampsia; failed induction of labor to end toxemia; maternal diabetes; maternal heart disease; placenta previa; Rh factor incompatibility; and renal disease.

Until quite recently, these probable indications were placed in the same category as mandatory ones. Changing trends, philosophies, and recent innovations in health care have made it possible for formerly inflexible rules to become more variable. It is imperative that health care providers, hospital policymakers and parents remember that individual considerations are the deciding factors. There are no hard and fast rules in these situations.

Active Genital Herpes. Herpes simplex II is a viral infection that may be transmitted to the baby as it passes through the birth canal. Active lesions in the birth passage or on the genitals at the time of birth can seriously infect the baby and cause brain damage, blindness, even death. If you have active genital herpes at the time of delivery or proven asymptomatic shedding (that is, no symptoms are experienced but the shedding is determined by laboratory testing), there is no negotiating: you must have a cesarean in order to protect the baby from risk. However, just because you have had herpes in the past does not necessarily mean that you must have a cesarean.

Eclampsia. Eclampsia is a sudden convulsive seizure without loss of consciousness during pregnancy or childbirth. Great strides have been made in treating eclampsia and toxemia (distribution of bacterial toxins through the blood stream). Individual circumstances and the predisposition of your doctor influence the method of delivery you will have. Severe cases of chronic hypertension (excessively high blood pressure) or toxemia may result in the need for a cesarean. Recent research shows that babies of such very ill mothers are often better off being delivered early, rather than remaining in the uterus.

Failed Induction of Labor to End Toxemia. If a mother-to-be is toxemic, the doctor may be inclined to induce labor artificially in order to deliver the compromised fetus whose well-being could be enhanced by early delivery. If induction of labor fails, a cesarean may be necessary (see page 27).

Maternal Diabetes. It used to be that women with diabetes were often unable to carry to term, much less have anything to say about which way their babies were delivered. Previously even normal pregnancies in diabetic women led to intrauterine fetal death.

Although maternal mortality associated with diabetes is now rare, if you are a diabetic mother, try to go to a special-pregnancy clinic. Usually found in large teaching hospitals, special-pregnancy clinics concern themselves with women whose pregnancies may be clouded by their medical conditions.

A diabetic mother can do much to help ensure the good outcome of her pregnancy and determine the method of delivery. For example, she must be meticulous in following her special diet during her entire pregnancy and be certain that her insulin levels are balanced. Cesarean rates for diabetic mothers are still high, but new methods of treatment and monitoring during pregnancy and improved newborn care have resulted in a decrease in the number of cesareans and diabetes-related birth problems.

Maternal Heart Disease. This is one of those indications that falls between mandatory and probable. Women with severe heart disease are currently enjoying the benefits of modern medicine and have a good chance of a positive outcome. However, there may still be complications in such instances. For example, pregnancy may place too great a strain upon the woman's heart and vascular system. On a reassuring note, cases have been cited where even women with heart valve implants now give birth to healthy babies.

As with diabetes and other maternal conditions, it's advantageous, if you have heart disease, to have your pregnancy guided by the help of a special-pregnancy clinic. If you cannot, you certainly should be treated by both a cardiologist and an obstetrician. Be sure to tell your heart doctor if you are planning to or have become pregnant. Medications, for example, may have to be changed or their dosage compensated for in light of your condition.

Placenta Previa. Placenta previa, although listed and explained under mandatory indications, is included here as well because it is sometimes possible, providing the placenta is only partially covering the cervix, to have a vaginal delivery.

Rh Factor Incompatibility and Renal Disease. With modern early diagnosis and treatment, Rh factor incompatibility is no longer as common as it once was. A cesarean delivery based solely upon Rh incompatibility is extremely rare. And renal (kidney) disease is now treated with sophisticated medical methods and thus is an infrequent—and not always inevitable—indication for surgical birth.

RELATIVE OR POSSIBLE INDICATIONS

Relative indications comprise at least 75 *percent* of all cesareans being done today. These indications are the most controversial, the most vague in medical definition and interpretation, and the most frequently avoidable. Not surprisingly, these indications are also the most potentially iatrogenic. Iatrogenic means a disease or problem created by an action or attitude of the physician. In other words, interventions into normal labor and delivery sometimes introduce complications which otherwise would not have occurred.

If a previous cesarean was performed for any one or a combination of the reasons below, then there is a 50 percent chance your cesarean may have been avoided, and you stand an excellent chance (providing you can find a cooperative doctor and hospital) of attempting subsequent vaginal delivery.

The possible/relative indications include: breech presentation; dystocia; CPD and fetopelvic disproportion; failed induction; failure to progress; fetal distress; multiple births (twins, triplets, etc.); postmature baby; premature and low birth weight babies; previous cesarean delivery; and special circumstances of the very young and more mature mother.

Breech Presentation. The ideal way for a baby to be positioned at the time of birth is with the head facing toward the mother's back and well down into the mother's pelvis. An increasingly common—and controversial—indication for cesarean delivery is breech presentation. A breech birth is one in which the baby comes out bottom or legs first (the parts usually covered by "breeches" or pants).

Not all breech-positioned babies are or should be delivered by cesarean. As Dr. P. R. Myerscough, author of *Munro Kerr's Operative Obstetrics,* states:

> Numerous reviews of breech delivery over the years have stressed the seriousness of this type of delivery

for the infant. Indeed, some of the *avant garde* have leaped to the conclusion that breech delivery is rarely, if ever, justifiable [vaginally], and should be entirely replaced by caesarean section, a view that I have to regard as ill-considered extremism.

. . .

I am thus led to conclude that caesarean section needs to be employed in a more selective way in cases of breech presentation, reserving the operation for those situations where the excess fetal mortality associated with vaginal delivery is high enough to justify the increased maternal risk.

. . .

Balancing the fetal and maternal interests (and this is what obstetrics is about) I believe an overall caesarean section rate of about 25–30% is prudent when the breech presents, with higher rates for the preterm breech.[1]

The rationale for delivering breech babies by cesarean is the fear that an attempted vaginal delivery (especially in a woman giving birth for the first time, and who thus has an untested pelvic outlet) will result in anoxia (cutting off or reduction of supply of oxygen to the fetus) or premature respiration of the baby before he or she is fully delivered. There is also the possibility that the baby's head may be too large to pass through the birth canal. Many doctors say that to avoid subjecting the baby to the possibility that the head will get stuck after the rest of the body has been delivered, they will not even consider vaginal delivery as an option.

Breech presentation occurs in approximately 3–4 percent of all births, and in 6–8 percent of pregnancies in which the mother is age thirty or older. It is also increasing among the very young (i.e., teenagers). Yet only in the past decade has breech presentation become miscategorized as an almost absolute indication for cesarean delivery. This means that many doctors who have been in practice for a number of years have become so accustomed to automatically delivering breeches by

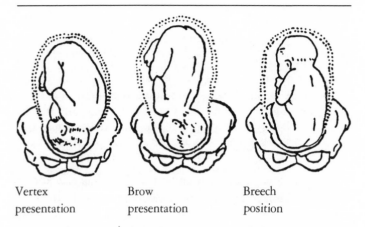

| Vertex | Brow | Breech |
| presentation | presentation | position |

cesarean that their skills for successfully performing a vaginal breech delivery have become somewhat rusty. Younger doctors who trained during the recent cesarean epidemic may have little or no training in how to attend a vaginal breech delivery. All too often, medical professionals simply assume that any baby who presents feet or buttocks first has to be delivered by cesarean. This is clearly not so. (It is also important to note that because breech babies are more likely to be premature, two instead of one relative or possible indications for cesarean delivery must be taken into consideration by birth attendants.)

The position of your baby can be determined early in pregnancy—long before labor begins—by the doctor or pre-natal care provider. This determination can be based on something as simple and old-fashioned as palpating (feeling) your abdomen during a routine prenatal visit and/or with use of ultrasound (if indicated). It's a good idea to ask what position your baby is in starting in the latter part of your second trimester and during the third trimester visits. Bear in mind, however, that lots of babies are breech for a while before labor starts and will automatically turn on their own. If yours doesn't, don't panic. You can probably rotate the baby to a head-down position simply and with minimal risk, either by yourself and/or with a doctor's aid.

To rotate a breech: If you know your baby is in the breech position and it is after the thirty-second week of pregnancy (up to which time many babies are breech and will shortly turn by themselves), by all means, start doing the *pelvic tilt.* It's a simple enough thing to do, takes very little time, can often be successful in rotating a breech, and is well worth the little effort it takes to very possibly protect yourself and your baby from a cesarean.

Using pillows, elevate your pelvis nine to twelve inches above your head while lying on the floor or another secure hard surface. Or, prop up an ironing board at one end so that you can lie on it with your head down. Wear an exercise leotard or loose, comfortable clothing. *Be sure you have an empty stomach* (even so, there's one side-effect you may experience: shortness of breath). Twice a day for ten minutes each time, recline on the floor and pillows or ironing board and imaging that your baby is turning while you bring one leg at a time in toward your abdomen. Holding your knee in your hands will help you bring your leg as close to your abdomen as possible. If this is uncomfortable for you, or if you want to alternate, you may also try supporting yourself on the floor on your hands and knees and bringing each leg individually up toward your abdomen/chest area.

If your baby still stubbornly refuses to turn, more and more doctors are now revising an older but proven effective method called external version. External version, simply, is the gentle rotation of your baby while still in utero from a breech position to a vertex presentation. All the mother has to do is to relax as much as possible—the more relaxed, the better. Some doctors use analgesics or uterine relaxants to aid relaxation and/or first do an ultrasound to determine the exact location of baby and placenta. Dr. Brooks Ranney, one doctor who has had wonderful success with external version, says that "the physician's attitude is as important as technique. . . . This is no place for a hasty or domineering approach, which is futile, and possibly dangerous. If the fetus cannot be turned forward, then it may be turned backward. If not today, then probably at the next office visit."[2]

A baby's being in the breech position at the time of labor certainly should not contraindicate vaginal delivery. However, in such instances, it is advised that the laboring woman have no interventions and ward off potential problems by *not* laboring on her back. There are various alternative positions for labor: squatting, semi-squatting (with someone supporting your arms and body from behind), standing, kneeling, hunkering on all fours or in a knee-chest position—or any combination of these as long as you feel comfortable. Change positions when you can't maintain one position any longer.

There's another key to achieving a successful vaginal delivery with a breech: there must be an environment that (at least until vaginal delivery of breeches again becomes the norm) exudes confidence about and belief in the natural processes of birth, even under unusual circumstances. The mother must have confidence in herself. Her birth attendant/coach must have confidence both in the laboring woman and in nature, and extra encouragement, verbal soothing, and pep talks are often required. The trickiest part, however, is having a doctor and support staff around you who also keep calm, have faith, and feel secure in themselves and in the natural variations and progressions of birth, and whose actions and words enhance the mother's natural ability. Not everyone attending a birth is a positive thinker, an optimist, or supportive. If a doctor, nurse, or other attendant sends out messages—whether stated or through body language and attitude—that they are clearly skeptical, if not downright convinced, that attempted vaginal birth with a breech cannot be safely accomplished, they will pass these fears on to the laboring woman. She, in turn, may have started out believing she could accomplish a safe vaginal delivery despite the odds, but the resistance she encounters may cause even the strongest to become discouraged. Her mind or her body may give up trying to buck the system.

For a breech baby who can't or won't be turned, and especially if this is a first baby, a routine cesarean delivery is the current medical fad. Let us hope it soon goes out of vogue. Doctors will argue that you're risking your baby's life if you don't submit to a cesarean. You'll suffocate it, they'll tell you. If this is your first baby, they will argue that your pelvis is untested and that they cannot be sure that you *could* get a baby out vaginally. The consensus will be that you really *have* to have a cesarean.

If you do have to have a cesarean (because you can't find a cooperative doctor with the skill and experience to allow for a trial of labor), then by all means insist at least on spontaneous labor. A scheduled primary or repeat cesarean without benefit of labor is often an invitation to Respiratory Distress Syndrome (RDS), which means that the baby's breathing systems are too immature to function properly outside the uterus. RDS is discussed more fully on page 85. Routinely scheduling cesareans in advance (with or without the results of antenatal tests to determine fetal maturity and well-being, even in women who know almost to the minute when they conceived) is convenient for the doctor and hospital but not necessarily beneficial to you or your baby. Remember: You are paying the doctor's fee for services rendered. Be sure your doctor is rendering the type, kind, and quality of service you want.

Dystocia. Dystocia refers to a difficult or abnormal labor. This is one of those catchall phrases that is open to much discussion and even more debate. In the strictest terms, dystocia refers to a labor that clearly fails to progress—when the cervix fails to dilate to the full 10 centimeters necessary for vaginal delivery and when contractions don't do the work they were intended to. Unfortunately, childbirth that isn't accomplished in the time span doctors think it should be from the onset of labor (though many women don't know exactly when their labors began) to actual delivery is often termed dystocia. An impatient doctor or one who arbitrarily sets a time limit for labor based upon personal or professional preferences may resort to a cesarean.

If you're in labor (beginning, middle, or after many hours have elapsed) and you're told they'll have to do a cesarean for dystocia, try any or all of the following measures.

Cesarean prevention measures: In most cases, there's no such thing as a dire emergency cesarean. Before you agree to an emergency, repeat, or elective cesarean, there is almost always time to take precautions that may avert the need for a cesarean.

1. An easy thing to do is to change the position in which you've been laboring. Whatever it is you've been doing, do something else. If you've been lying down, get up and walk around. Or turn on your left side and prop yourself up with pillows all around. Squat. Sit on a birthing stool. Get up on your hands and knees, perhaps even do the pelvic rock from this position (see p. 43). It's gratifying to know that many labors are often stimulated and the quality of the contractions improved by simply altering position.

2. If your membranes are still intact, take a nice long bath. If your membranes are ruptured, take a shower instead. If you happen to be in a situation where neither a bath nor a shower is possible, or if you don't feel up to it, put warm compresses on your abdomen or use a not-too-hot water bottle or heating pad.

3. Sluggish labors are often vastly improved with gentle nipple stimulation since this helps release your body's natural hormone oxytocin. You can also release this natural labor stimulant by achieving orgasm. Intercourse with penetration, however, may not feel comfortable or be advisable under the circumstances, particularly after membranes have ruptured. It is also difficult if not impossible to achieve orgasm in a hospital environment where there is no privacy. A labor that

has turned sluggish will greatly benefit from your efforts to revive it naturally. Don't forget: If you don't at least try to help yourself, you may well be given the drug Pitocin which is a synthetic version of your body's own supply of oxytocin.

4. There is nothing better to ease tension and help you relax than the verbal encouragement of your husband, labor coach, or the delivery staff. A back or leg rub may also be useful.

5. To this day, many hospital policies banish nourishment for laboring women. Should anesthesia be necessary, they argue (and as we know, anesthesia is not always optional in traditional hospitals but mandatory and inevitable for most birthing women), the woman who had recently eaten might throw up and choke on vomit. Aspiration pneumonia (i.e., blockage of breathing passages from ingested foods) is the medical term for this condition. But if anesthesia were necessary, even general anesthesia, modern medicine has ways of making sure that nobody dies on the table from aspiration of vomitus. Labor is hard work and requires that you have nourishment in order to carry on with it efficiently, thus reducing your risk of needing a cesarean. Even marathon runners drink to replenish their fluids and add calories for the long haul. You should be able at least to have fluids—milk, juice, soup, or broth. In fact, you may not even feel like eating solid foods. If the hospital you're in won't allow anything other than ice chips and/or lollipops, then by all means maintain and replace your body's fluid loss with ice chips, lots and lots of ice chips. Although they contain high amounts of sugar, a few lollipops won't hurt either.

6. In lieu of the prescription drugs (which can inhibit labor) that hospitals order for laboring women in pain, you might want to try calcium tablets to promote muscle tone and maintain strong muscular contractions. Adele Davis suggests taking a small quantity of vitamin D to aid calcium absorption.

7. If your obstetrician tells you during labor that you must have a cesarean due to fetal distress (covered later in this chapter), make it your business or the business of your husband or labor attendant to find out first how serious the degree of fetal distress is. Did your baby's heartrate take a dramatic, life-threatening and irremedial plunge? If so, then a cesarean seems to be indicated. Changes in fetal heartrates are sometimes harmless swings in the fetal heart pattern; variations may correct themselves with time and/or a change in the mother's position. These non-threatening changes in fetal heartrate can, however, cause a doctor to perform a cesarean too hastily and unnecessarily since the fear of being sued for malpractice prompts the unfounded diagnosis of fetal distress. If this is a dire emergency, then a quick cesarean may be the only way to correct the situation of a baby whose well-being is truly endangered. Before consenting to a cesarean, it is best for mother and baby to have someone acting on their behalf question the diagnosis.

8. Sometimes you have to convince yourself that you don't want any drugs during labor since the effect of almost all medications contributed to the cesarean epidemic. Not only may these drugs inhibit labor but they'll cross the placenta and affect your baby, too. Prepare a "Birth Requests" list long before you go into labor. Talk it over with your doctor in advance. Take it with you to the hospital. Refer to it if you feel yourself faltering. Post another copy on the labor room door or wall above your bed. Then, when you go into labor, you'll be less likely to accept medicines and other interventions that the hospital staff, with all the best intentions, often feel it's their duty to recommend. Be sure to let your coach know what you want so that if you are not up to defending your anti-interference preference in the midst of a set of strong contractions, that person is designated to work on your behalf. Obviously, though, if you've passed the point of your endurance, you should not feel guilty about accepting medication.

9. Have you considered staying at home for as long as possible during labor before going to the hospital? The longer you avoid going to the hospital, the more able you may be to avoid interventions and possibly a cesarean delivery.

10. Have you considered staying home to have your baby in order to prevent any and all interventions into birth, as many more parents now seem to be doing? If so, make sure yours is a thoroughly prepared and well-thought-through home birth plan.

CPD (Cephalopelvic Disproportion) and Fetopelvic Disproportion. "Cephalo" refers to the head size of the fetus. "Feto" refers to the overall size of the fetal body. If you are told that your baby is too large to pass through the pelvic outlet, this means that your cesarean was performed because of CPD. When is a baby too large to pass through the pelvic outlet? Each case must be judged individually. However, this diagnosis is a very common one today, and suspiciously frequent at a time when the average birth weight of today's babies has risen only a few ounces. How can there be so many diagnoses of CPD when mothers are not getting any smaller—in fact, the average height for American women is slowly increasing—and babies are not getting much bigger?

In Chapter 5, "Tests to Determine Fetal Maturity and Well-being," methods of determining the size of the fetus in relationship to the size of the mother's pelvis are discussed, as well as their unreliability as an infallible guideline. Some women are able to deliver ten-pound babies vaginally. In fact, one of my best high school friends waited until she was in her thirties to have two children. The first weighed over 8 pounds, the second, almost 13. She delivered both vaginally—despite the fact that, in addition to what was diagnosed during her second pregnancy as a very large baby, Jeri also had placental problems!

There are times when CPD truly is a problem. There are times when there are spatial or positional problems, or both.

However, CPD will be less often (mis)diagnosed when American medicine relies less on machines and intervention, and regains a more relaxed attitude toward the time element of labor, and reassesses what constitutes abnormal labor and true cephalopelvic disproportion. Although doctors may order x-rays during pregnancy or labor to determine CPD, these are *not* reliable tools upon which to base a diagnosis—not to mention the fact that they are potentially dangerous to the unborn baby. To avoid a cesarean, in the case of CPD, all you may need is more time or a change of position (squatting is especially recommended).

If there is a question about whether or not your baby will be born vaginally, what will probably happen is that you will go into labor and your labor will be monitored closely. In the absence of progress, or in the presence of fetal distress, a cesarean may be indicated. Beware that CPD may not be suspected until after labor has progressed for some time. CPD is often a surprise to both the expectant mother and the obstetrician.

Each woman and each of her pregnancies should be judged on an individual basis. Women who have had one or more vaginal deliveries may have CPD in subsequent pregnancies, although this is exceedingly uncommon. And as we have seen time and time again, women diagnosed as having pelvic outlets too small to deliver their first baby or babies successfully deliver even larger babies in subsequent VBAC births.

Failed Induction. Induction of labor via drugs (Pitocin) and/or surgically rupturing membranes is usually relatively safe and successful, but can be associated with complications. Should vaginal delivery follow artificial induction, many of the same problems are encountered as with scheduled cesareans: babies may be born with Respiratory Distress Syndrome (RDS). Artificial induction of labor, either at the mother's request or the physician's, was far too common in the 1940s and 1950s. Artificially inducing labor was a trend of that era based on convenience rather than medical necessity. We know enough now, at least, to have banned the use of Pitocin to electively induce labor for mere convenience.

Diabetes and toxemia are two substantial, medically sound reasons for trying to initiate labor in some instances. Remaining in utero in these cases often is more of a danger to the baby than early delivery and intensive neonatal care. Should rupture of the membranes and/or the introduction of Pitocin fail to induce labor, a cesarean will be performed.

Once a woman's membranes have ruptured or been ruptured for her, it is presumed she is at great risk of infection. What surprises many is that a not-so-old medical theory held that such infection would occur (if it was going to) within a seventy-two-hour time frame. Germs must be getting more aggressive today since, without explanation, and even when no signs of infection present themselves, cesareans are often performed within twelve to twenty-four hours after rupture.

Fetal Distress. Modern fetal monitors are both a blessing and a curse. In the past decade, it has become common to monitor the fetus while a woman is in labor. During labor and before the membranes have ruptured, belts are placed around the woman's abdomen to chart contractions and fetal heart rate. Once the membranes have ruptured (or been ruptured), a tiny electrode may be inserted vaginally and pushed into the fetus's scalp. The good intention behind the widespread use of this machine in today's hospitals is quite simple: checking the baby's progress in utero (i.e., making sure the unborn child is getting a sufficient supply of oxygen and is otherwise unendangered) was originally intended for use in high-risk labors. Now it's used on almost every woman who checks into a hospital to have her baby (there are exceptions, notably enlightened conventional labor and delivery units and many Normal Birth Centers and Alternative Birth Centers). Electronic fetal monitors free up the amount of time a hospital staff must spend providing one-on-one time. If properly inserted (a big "if"), there is little or no need to go from bed to bed checking each woman's progress with a fetoscope (a stethoscope to hear the fetal heart) at frequent intervals. Instead, computerized information is sent from the body of the laboring woman through a maze of electronic wires to the bank of screens at a central station, or at least to a print-out, which, like ticker tape, grows longer and longer.

Has increased use of the fetal monitor led to an improvement in fetal outcome? No, it has not.

If you are not yet familiar with electronic fetal monitors, they are machines that chart both uterine contractions and fetal heart rate. These are recorded continuously onto graphs. The attending physician, nurse, or midwife reads the chart and interprets what it indicates. When a potentially threatening change in the pattern of the fetal heart is noted, or if contractions become prolonged or markedly irregular, a cesarean may be necessary. Then again, it may not. For examples of things a laboring woman can do to help prevent cesareans, see pages 23 to 26 in this chapter.

An ominous change in the fetal heartbeat is called fetal distress, which should not be confused with the ordinary, non-threatening and usually transitory stress which the unborn baby undergoes during normal labor. Ominous changes, however, (indicated by the data from the fetal monitor and/or when meconium [fetal excrement] is present) mean that the supply of oxygen to the baby may be endangered and/or that the baby may be aspirating (inhaling) meconium. Thus, a cesarean delivery may be founded on a very real need to get the baby out as quickly and safely as possible.

Prior to the introduction of electronic fetal monitors, the means of determining the fetal heart rate in utero was by using fetoscopes or standard stethoscopes. Oddly enough, as wonderful as many high-tech innovations are, routine electronic fetal monitoring may not be one of the best of them since studies have shown that when fetal monitoring is compared with "old-fashioned" ausculation (manual affirmation of the baby's heart rate), there is no difference in terms of fetal outcome. But in terms of the cesarean rate, there is a marked difference. There are more cesareans!

There is and will continue to be a great deal of discussion among medical and lay persons about the use and/or abuse of fetal monitoring. Fears that the monitor will mesmerize the hospital staff and the father are not unfounded. In addition, fetuses that are monitored can suffer scalp bleeding, abscesses, and even punctures in the parts of the body other than the bony part of its head (as can happen if the electrode is mistakenly placed). Mothers, too, are at greater risk of infection.

In high-risk labors, fetal monitoring can be a blessing. Yet there does not seem to be any great advantage in monitoring *all* laboring women (although numerous disadvantages have come to light). An experienced midwife, nurse, or doctor can check fetal progress just as surely with a fetoscope—although not as conveniently *for them.*

There is another consideration: things can go wrong with machines. It happens all the time, every day, at home and at work, and just because the machine in question happens to be in a hospital does not mean that it is immune to malfunction. It is possible that a monitor indicates fetal distress not because the fetus is experiencing distress, but because of mechanical malfunction. What is more, human error and misinterpretation also add to the possibility of misdiagnosed fetal distress.

When you are attached to a fetal monitor, you may have to lie flat on your back and keep still in order to get an accurate reading. This is not so with newer machines which allow some freedom of movement and permit the mother to choose between lying flat on her back, lying on her side, or sitting up in bed. As we know, lying flat on your back during labor creates pressure (and thus problems) on the vena cava (the major vein running from the lower extremities) which often results in a compromised oxygen supply to both mother and unborn baby.

Again, this is a situation in which the suggestions found on pages 23 to 26 can make the difference between a cesarean for fetal distress and a vaginal delivery.

The *judicious* use of fetal monitors has its benefits under special circumstances, but it should not be routine or a requirement.

Multiple Births. If you're expecting twins or triplets, you may wonder if it's essential that you give birth to them by cesarean. The answer is maybe. Individual circumstances and who you've chosen for a doctor as well as where you'll be giving birth influence the method of delivery. It takes extra skill to safely deliver more than one baby at a time, by either method. Advances in newborn care, which are much greater than at any time previously, play a significant role in making sure multiple births result in healthy babies.

Postmature Baby. Pregnancy usually lasts about forty weeks. There is always some variation. However, when a woman has not gone into labor spontaneously after the forty-second week, the baby may be postmature (overdue). It has been customary in such cases to try to induce labor with an intravenous drip of Pitocin and/or artificial rupture of membranes. Trying to induce labor is rather like trying to jump-start a car's battery. Sometimes it works, and sometimes it doesn't.

If you're a few days past your due date and everything else is normal (and let us remember that nature has the cards stacked in favor of normal pregnancy, labor, and delivery), there is little if any cause for alarm. But if your pregnancy has gone on longer than normal, then the placenta, which is the lifeline for the baby, may start to function less adequately, thus compromising the baby's well-being.

The placenta is designed by nature to function for a certain period of time. There are variations, and a few record-breaking pregnancies have come out all right. If you are two weeks or more overdue, this does not necessarily mean that your baby is postmature. What it may mean is that the date of conception and estimated due date were inaccurate. Also, there is some leeway with regard to average gestational duration. But if there is a question about postmaturity, chances are good that your doctor will either attempt to induce labor and/or will employ antenatal tests to determine fetal maturity and well-being. In these tests, which are covered in Chapter 5, it is possible to determine while the baby is still in utero if everything is functioning properly or if there is a need to intervene in order to prevent possible postmaturity problems by scheduling the delivery before the onset of spontaneous labor. It is your responsibility to decide if you wish to undergo these tests.

Premature and Low Birth Weight Babies. It is not yet irrefutably known if premature babies and those of low birthweight are actually better off being born by cesarean. Into this category we must also place multiple birth babies since they sometimes are both premature and of low birth weight. There are improved survival rates among these babies, but this may be due more to improved peri- and neonatal care than to the method of delivery. There is still great debate over whether it is safer and better for such babies to be delivered by cesarean or to be subjected to the possible "stresses" of normal vaginal labor and delivery. Nancy Edwards Dow, M.D., a neonatologist on the staff of U.S.C. Women's Hospital in Los Angeles, offered this comment in an April, 1985 interview: "There is a lot of very soft work but very good work being done now at our hospital which shows that low birth weight babies delivered by cesarean have a better chance of surviving."

Previous Cesarean Delivery. Once considered an automatic indication for a repeat cesarean, this is no longer the case. For a thorough discussion, see Chapter 16, page 223.

Special Circumstances of the Very Young and More Mature Mothers. There are more and more mothers over thirty and under twenty than ever before. It is assumed that their pregnancies and deliveries are more difficult to manage than those of their counterparts of "ideal" childbearing age, that is, women in their twenties. Mature mothers (those over thirty) are regarded as having "premium" pregnancies, which means that they haven't as many years left to procreate and thus great value is placed (as well it should be for a woman of any age) on ensuring an optimal outcome. It is also broadly generalized medically that all older mothers are at higher risk than any other age group except teenagers.

The story behind teenage pregnancies (sometimes referred to as "children having children") is a sad and alarming one. The teenage mother is quite different from the woman who postpones childbearing until she is in her thirties or forties. The common factor is that both teens and mature mothers are *assumed* to encounter greater risks. Christopher Norwood writes: "The course of labor of 'older' mothers—variously defined as over age thirty, thirty-five or forty—has not been well researched. Probably not more than twenty studies in the past twenty years have attempted to define whether 'elderly primigravidas'— the tasteless medical term for older women having a first birth—are at special risk. (By contrast, the available research on breech deliveries, which constitute only 4 percent of births, would fill a library shelf.)"[3]

It is essential that "special" mothers search and find doctors who will treat their pregnancies with an open mind rather than with a preordained bias. They—and you—should give the benefit of doubt in your favor that you will be able to have a perfectly normal, uncomplicated pregnancy, labor, and delivery. Dr. Nancy Edwards Dow, herself a mother who had children in her mid-thirties, says, "To be perfectly factual, I chose the best obstetrical care I could find, although I didn't give birth in an NBC [Normal Birth Center] or ABC [Alternative Birth Center] because they weren't available at the time. I was definitely concerned about totally unnecessary intervention. I was in labor with Mary for six hours. With Mark, because of my blood pressure, they wanted to do a cesarean. So what I did was to have him in only two hours—before they had time. I was determined I was not going to have a c-section."

The predictions of the dire consequences when a woman

chooses not to accept every obstetrical dictum and caution sometimes have a very odd twist to them. When a health care provider suggests or implies that it is essential to use every intervention available in order to have a good outcome, the portents of what will befall anyone who refuses them may actually become self-fulfilling prophecies. Even when you start off with great self-confidence and the courage of your convictions, the power of suggestion—particularly when it is encountered with each prenatal visit and each hospital mailing outlining its policies and procedures—may undermine you. You may end up thinking more about the perils of childbirth than on your innate ability to have a normal birth. This, in turn, can profoundly affect the outcome of your pregnancy, labor, and method of delivery. In other words, even if you are not of the so-called ideal childbearing age, this does not mean that you will automatically encounter problems and require surgical delivery in order to have a healthy baby.

REASSURANCE

If you must have a cesarean on account of an absolute indication, your doctor will almost always be aware of this during your pregnancy and should inform you. This way you'll be able to prepare for the birth, get your body in shape so that you'll be in the best possible physical condition for the rigors of surgery and caring for a newborn. If you have a probable indication, read everything you can find on the subject of labor and delivery to determine what you can do to avert a cesarean. For the possible/relative category of indications, it's always better to know too much than too little in preparation.

When the decision is made to do a cesarean delivery, it is important to remember that a number of factors are taken into account. Each pregnancy, each mother, and each baby is different. The indications should always be judged (but are not) on an individual basis, taking into account the mother's medical history, the progress of labor, dilation of the cervix, possible signs of fetal distress (and what might be done to rectify them before they lead to an otherwise preventable cesarean), and other conditions that may make it necessary to deliver a baby as quickly and safely as possible.

If your baby is delivered by cesarean, it is important to bear in mind that you are *not* a failure. Having a baby is not a challenge to your femininity, nor is it a game of Russian roulette. A healthy baby and a positive birth experience for the family are the most important considerations. Cesarean childbirth, despite those who say otherwise, sometimes does have advantages that outweigh its disadvantages. With these words, remember, too, that I allow for far more flexibility and take into consideration many factors some authors ignore. If you have done everything in your power to avoid a cesarean, you should not feel as though you have not only disappointed yourself but failed your "sisters."

Cesarean section, because it is major surgery, is more risky than vaginal delivery. But if you have to have a cesarean, you will most likely be safe and your infant will also be healthy. As recently as forty years ago, the prospect of a mother's surviving a cesarean was slim; but tremendous strides have been made that ensure the survival and well-being of both mother and baby. As we saw in the preceding chapter, some babies *are* given a better opportunity to thrive than they might have under adverse vaginal birthing conditions.

In summary, avoid a cesarean whenever possible, even if it means you have to put out additional effort in finding a cooperative doctor and birthing place. These efforts will not go unrewarded. But if you must become a parent via cesarean, give yourself some credit and reflect on the fact that cesarean childbirth is not only relatively safe but sometimes unavoidable.

THE CESAREAN MOTHER: WHO IS SHE?

Rampant in contemporary folklore is the image of a typical cesarean mother. She is supposed to be short, small-boned, perhaps frail and nervous. Some people claim that tiny feet betray the woman who must have a cesarean, others that it is a pointed jaw or thin lips. All elderly primigravidas (women having their first child after age thirty or thirty-five) are supposed to need a cesarean delivery. Just as women who have irregular painful periods were, until very recently, erroneously blamed for bringing this upon themselves, so, too, women who are uncomfortable in their roles as childbearers are often blamed for imposing cesarean deliveries upon themselves. The only generalization that can be made about the typical cesarean woman is that she comes in all sizes, shapes, ages, and from every ethnic and socioeconomic background. With new, sophisticated tests of fetal maturity and well-being, and because the cesarean procedure is now a safe alternative to a complicated birth the number of cesareans is rising. Along with this increase, the kinds of women who have cesarean births have come to include almost any childbearer—even mothers who have had one or more vaginal deliveries.

There is nothing "abnormal" or "wrong" with the cesarean woman. If all women under five feet tall had to have cesareans, there would be no other way of giving birth in countries such as India, Pakistan, China, and Japan, where almost all the women are short by American standards. This is not to say that American women under five feet tall are excluded from the list of those who have cesarean deliveries. An early 1960s study reported in a medical journal indicated that of 117 women under five feet, a slightly higher percentage did have cesarean births. Women who are almost six feet tall may sometimes require an abdominal delivery. Happy, feminine women who produce many children by choice may need to deliver by this alternative means. Socialites, welfare recipients, single mothers, career women, factory workers, doctoral candidates, eighth grade drop-outs—anyone may have a cesarean. The point is that the cesarean mother is anyone. Who delivers by cesarean is less a matter of the mother's physique than of the baby's position, general condition, or gestational maturation.

However, before we become too accepting of the high incidence of cesareans, please note what "An Evaluation of Cesarean Section in the United States," published by the U.S. Department of Health, Education and Welfare in 1979,[4] had to say about the most likely candidates for surgical delivery. The dichotomies here are too obvious and follow too many curious coincidences for us to say that there is no rhyme or reason behind the current high incidence. For example, this report tells us that some of the most likely candidates for surgical delivery are highly educated women, college graduates being more likely than any group of women except those with the least amount of education. Well-to-do women and very poor women are more likely than the middle economic group to have cesareans. The youngest mothers (teenagers) and oldest mothers are more prone to giving birth by surgical means. So, too, are the diverse populace having either the most comprehensive private medical insurance or public insurance. Oddly enough, the cesarean rate is also influenced by what type of hospital a woman goes to for birth: both the woman who goes to a private hospital and the woman who gives birth at a clinic are more likely to have cesareans. The only thing that is *not* surprising about this study is that the most likely candidate for a cesarean section is still the woman who has already had one or more previous cesareans.

For a discussion of the possibilities, risks, benefits, and advantages of subsequent vaginal delivery, please see Chapters 5, 15 and 16.

PREGNANCY

Almost without exception, the cesarean pregnancy progresses in the same way as the pregnancies of women who deliver vaginally. The cesarean mother experiences the same anticipations, joys, trepidations, and physical sensations shared by others. Questions common to all expectant couples arise: Will our baby be all right? Will pregnancy and birth affect our relationship? Will we be able to do the same things we used to? How can we support a family financially?

Pregnancy is a time of emotional ambivalence. The pregnant woman is very vulnerable. She experiences mood swings that confound her. She may be ecstatic about the baby growing inside of her most of the time. At other times, she may tearfully wonder why she thought getting pregnant was a good idea in the first place. Not only does the body change but the hormonal balance is shifted, so that a pregnant woman sometimes feels as though she is on an emotional roller coaster. One minute she is as happy as a clam; the next, she may be in tears over the most trivial incident. Physical changes put her off balance, too, both literally and figuratively. When a woman is pregnant, she is pregnant from the ends of her hair to the tips of her toes. Her whole body, not just the contents of her uterus, is involved. Those around her may find the changes as bewildering and hard to deal with as she does. Within seconds she can change from "benevolent earth mother" to "wicked witch." At times when she needs support and reassurance most, her attitude may make it difficult for those around her to give it. Pregnant women can be likened to porcupines: they're soft, loving, and in need of cuddling on the inside but occasionally present an exterior that makes it hard for anyone to get close. Pregnancy is a tumultuous time. The "couple" is to become a family. The woman is to become a mother, and she may feel that she has lost her "girlishness." Now is the time when she must "grow up," no matter how young or old she is when she has her first baby. Her relationships with the baby's father and future grandparents also change. The parents' greatest hopes and deepest fears come to the surface. Pregnancy and childbirth have social, economic, sexual, and individual implications. With so much to think about, pregnancy may be a time of stress for the couple, especially the mother, even if the baby is wanted and planned for.

The Role of the Father or Other Support Person. Cesarean delivery alters the father's role—but only slightly. During pregnancy the cesarean father will do the same things as any other expectant father: support his wife emotionally, attend prenatal visits to the obstetrician when possible, rub his wife's back, pitch in with the chores, help ready the baby's room and equipment, and participate in prenatal classes.

Because the newly delivered cesarean mother must have additional help, the father will play a key role in helping the family achieve the best possible start.

COPING WITH PHYSICAL DISCOMFORT

A number of minor but disconcerting conditions are associated with pregnancy. What can be done to relieve these problems? Here are some suggestions that may be helpful:

Heartburn. As the uterus grows, the entrance to the stomach can be pushed into the chest cavity, and this may cause heartburn. Instead of three big meals a day, try eating a number of small meals. Stuffing yourself with quantities of food at any one sitting will only aggravate the problem. Junk foods and fried or fatty foods will also increase the chances of heartburn. It is better to stand up or sit up for a while after eating. Reclining may make the condition worse.

Hot Flashes. During pregnancy there will be two extra pints of blood in your body, most of it in the uterus, and this extra blood adds additional heat to your body. When your body is too hot, cool it off. Warmish baths are good. Turning down the thermostat will save energy as well as keep you cooler. If you feel comfortable doing it, take your clothes off. If not, try wearing loose cotton garments. Underpants are unnecessary and may, if synthetic, increase the likelihood of vaginal infection—a condition to which pregnant women are prone. Cotton allows the skin to breathe. Rayon and other synthetics and blends do not allow for the free exchange of air. Bras can be discarded, too, unless the breasts are enlarged or uncomfortable.

Chest or Rib Pains. Pain or discomfort under the ribs or chest should be brought to your doctor's attention. (It is always a good idea to write down questions for the doctor when they come to mind. Keeping a special notebook handy is better than saving questions in your head. Unless you write them down as you think of them, you'll probably forget most of them when you are in the doctor's office). Pressure is probably caused by the fact that as the baby grows the chest expands sideways and some organs get pushed out of place. Some babies learn early that their mother's ribs are excellent for kicking and nudging. To cope, place your arms above your head and stretch out to the side opposite from where you're being kicked. Or, raise both hands over your head and reach for the sky.

Poor Circulation. Blood flows from the head, to the

heart, to the baby, and finally to the feet. As it returns it has a harder time getting back up. Elevate your feet on a pillow several times a day and at night to improve circulation. Also, lie on your left side.

Shortness of Breath. When a pregnant woman lies flat on her back, she invites shortness of breath because the weight of the uterus and baby are on the vena cava, the major vein going into the heart from the lower extremities. Lying flat on the back may also reduce the amount of oxygen mother and baby receive. As a general rule, never let the baby lie on you. It is permissible for you to lie on the baby. Women who never felt the urge to lie directly on their stomachs often crave sleeping this way during pregnancy. Go ahead if you want to: it won't hurt the baby, but it may be uncomfortable for you. Some women place twin beds together with a space in between just wide enough to accommodate their bellies, and lie with their head, shoulders, and chest on one bed, and their legs and feet on the other. Another (perhaps better) solution is to place a stack of pillows under your chest and hips. A foam block scooped out in the middle may also allow you to lie comfortably on your stomach. The best position is to lie on your *left* side, with pillows under your shoulders and between your legs, which should be slightly flexed at the knees.

Leg Cramps. Leg cramps are common during pregnancy. To relieve cramps in your legs or feet, place your feet against a wall or bed frame and push for a few seconds several times every day. If there is someone to help you, ask that they hold your foot firmly and press your toes toward your head until the cramp is relieved. Supplementing your diet with additional calcium from calcium tablets or calcium-rich foods (milk, cheese, leafy vegetables such as collard greens, kale, mustard and turnip greens) also helps reduce cramps and improve muscle tone and function. Calcium is also valuable in helping blood to clot, aiding the heart in functioning properly, and maintaining or building strong bones and teeth.

Extra Pigmentation. Patches of dark skin on the

body, and a line extending from the naval to the pelvic bone, are fairly common during pregnancy. There is little that can be done, but this extra pigmentation will clear up after the baby has been born. This extra coloration may serve to "toughen" the body in preparation for labor.

Stretch Marks. Either you get stretch marks or you don't. If your body is prone to stretch marks, you will get them no matter what you do. A good diet and exercise will help prevent them. Tight clothing aggravates the condition. Mineral oil is inexpensive and works just as well as costly creams and lotions. Use mineral oil in place of make-up remover, bath oil, or massage oil. It might even help those stretch marks a bit. Vitamins E and A may also help prevent stretch marks and dry skin. During pregnancy, it is best to check with your doctor before taking additional amounts of any vitamin or mineral supplement. Buy an aloe vera plant—nature's skin healer—and keep it outdoors or in a sunny window. Cut off part of a stalk, slit it lengthwise, and slather the sticky juice over stretch marks or burns. Aloe vera is gooey, but it is also extremely effective.

Sexuality. Some women discover that they are aroused more easily during pregnancy. This may be partially caused by hormonal changes, and perhaps it is also partly due to the new awareness and pride a woman may have in her changing body. Making love may seem freer and less complicated during pregnancy since birth control is unnecessary. Unless there are special medical contraindications, pregnant women can do anything they like in the way of making love. Always check with your doctor or midwife if you have questions. Few doctors now impose bans on intercourse during the first three months and the last six weeks of pregnancy as they used to—special cases excepted, which is why it's best to make certain that you have no restrictions.

The mother may want and need the expression of love during this time, and the father has the same needs and drives as ever. As the baby grows, the couple may discover that the "missionary" position of lovemaking is uncomfortable, especially for the mother. Pregnancy can be a time of exploration and experimentation with different positions, oral sex, and pleasures that can include or exclude penetration. The mother-to-be may enjoy the closeness and relaxation that lovemaking brings, but she may find that she does not always have to achieve orgasm to be fulfilled.

There are women who are "turned off" to lovemaking during pregnancy. In some cases, this may be an excuse a woman uses to keep her husband from "bothering" her. More commonly, however, it is caused by extra physical fatigue, the discomfort of the enlarged uterus, intermittent nausea, and other physical problems. Or, the mother may truly fear that making love will somehow damage or hurt the baby, especially if she has had a miscarriage or stillbirth. As always, she should check with her doctor.

Backache. Pregnant women are subject to backaches for two reasons: (1) that human beings have evolved into creatures who stand on two feet, rather than walking on four legs, and (2) that our machine age has almost totally eliminated tasks that require exercise. Backache will not be as frequent a problem if you stand up straight, tuck in your fanny (imagine that you are carrying a cork around in your bottom and you don't want it to fall out), and keep your shoulders back. Exercising and lifting properly by kneeling instead of bending from the waist also helps.

Tailor Sitting. Sit on the floor with your legs crossed at the ankles in a position similar to the yoga lotus position. Allow your shoulders to be slightly relaxed. This exercise helps to distribute the weight of the uterus in a more comfortable manner. It also promotes muscle tone in the pelvis and thighs. Squatting with the soles of both feet flat on the ground, if you can do it, is an excellent preparation for childbirth.

Pelvic Rock. The pelvic rock will help relieve

backache and promote muscle tone. It can be done standing up, or resting on your hands and knees on the floor, or lying on your back with knees bent.

To do the pelvic rock standing up, place one hand on your abdomen just below the bulge and the other hand on your lower back. Push your pelvis forward. Count slowly to three. Then push the pelvis back and hold to the count of three. Do this several times each day or whenever you have a backache.

The pelvic rock can be even more effective if you get down on your hands and knees either on the floor or on a firm bed. Push the pelvis forward, count slowly to three, and then arch only your hips and lower back, again counting to three. Often the relief will be immediate.

Pelvic-Floor Exercises (also known as Kegals). Maintaining muscle tone in the pelvic-floor area is important not only during pregnancy but throughout your adult life. The pelvic floor is the series of elastic muscles used in defecation, urination, and intercourse. They also support the uterus and fetus. If muscle tone is not maintained, a prolapsed uterus can result and cause backache or extreme pain. Lack of muscle tone can also lead to difficulty in muscle coordination during urination or defecation. Men are surprised to learn that they, too, have pelvic-floor muscles; if their muscles become lax, they may suffer from prostate and other problems.

Two exercises should be practiced daily. One is to imagine that you are holding a pencil in your vagina and "write" the numbers from 0 to 9 with the pencil. The second exercise is to pretend that your pelvic-floor muscles have become an elevator. Start at the first floor, then bring the elevator up to the second floor, and hold there to the count of ten. Bring the elevator up to the third, fourth, and fifth floors, stopping at each floor long enough to count to ten. Reverse the process until you are back on the first floor. Instead of stopping, plunge the elevator down one more floor into the basement. To complete the exercise, bring the elevator back up to the first floor and relax.

These exercises can be done inconspicuously anytime during the day. Some people do them while cleaning the house, watching television, sitting in the car waiting for a light to change, or whenever. They should be practiced several times a day. You may feel "clumsy" or "uncoordinated" when you first begin. With practice comes proficiency. In addition to promoting muscle tone, these exercises can be a boon to your sex life. Try them the next time you make love. If you haven't done them before, they will add an extra, interesting dimension to your lovemaking.

DRUGS

The editors of *Consumer Reports, "The Medicine Show,"* note that until the horrible thalidomide scandal of the early sixties, the medical community assumed that the placenta "was a sort of guardian angel, a St. Peter standing at the gates of the umbilical cord to let needed nutrients through while holding back harmful germs and chemicals. [German measles was one known exception.] . . . Rather than being a barrier to the transfer of drugs from the mother to the fetus, writes Dr. Virginia Apgar of the National Foundation–March of Dimes, 'the placenta is a sieve. Almost everything ingested by or injected into the mother can be expected to reach the fetus within a few minutes.' Alcohol, antibiotics, aspirins, barbiturates, sulfonamides and tranquilizers are but a few of the common, and possibly harmful, substances known to get through."[1] Catherine Milinaire in *Birth* further cautions that

> this includes harmful chemicals, soda pops, . . . or puffing any kind of smoke as a daily habit. . . . Most of the damage that occurs because of drugs happens during the first four months of pregnancy. At that

time some damage can occur to the baby's growth because the cells are being formed and the structure of the new person is developing. In later months, drugs could cause minor complications. The problem is that most women, even though they may know of their pregnancy during the early months, do not realize the extent of damage that can be caused by drugs. This is especially true at this early stage since you do not really feel or look pregnant. Yet it cannot be overemphasized that these are the most crucial months in the formation of the new being.[2]

Common sense and a wealth of easily obtainable information tells us that drugs—either prescription or over-the-counter—should be used only with the advice and consent of your obstetrician.

It is now acceptable in all but a few social and religious circles to drink. Will the *moderate* use of alcohol during pregnancy adversely affect the unborn baby? Probably not. In fact, a glass or two of wine with dinner may serve to relax the mother-to-be. Warm milk before bed may also help you to fall asleep.

By our own government's estimate, more than eighteen million people have tried marijuana. It stands to reason that among these millions, a few have been female and pregnant. What is the truth about marijuana and its effects on the fetus? No one knows the answer. You may have friends who have had perfectly healthy babies even though they smoke marijuana regularly, but no drug (including tobacco) is without potential danger to the consumer and the developing fetus.

Women who smoke marijuana or do any other kind of drug (uppers, downers, cocaine, LSD, etc.) should talk with their doctors, a drug therapist or a hot line counselor. Usually there is some hesitation because the expectant mother fears that the doctor will not understand, will disapprove, or will compound her guilt by telling her she will almost certainly give birth to a deformed or damaged baby. If you simply must smoke during pregnancy (either marijuana or cigarettes), or if you take any other kind of drug, bear in mind that all drugs in all quantities may have an adverse effect on you and your unborn baby. If you cannot give up your indulgences, it may be helpful if you keep the indulgence to a bare minimum, scrupulously maintain a well-balanced diet, take prenatal vitamins regularly, and get adequate rest and exercise. One of the problems is that drugs deplete the body's supply of essential nutrients and create an additional drain on energy reserves and the body's ability to avoid or fight infection.

If you would like to wean yourself from any kind of drug, medical advice and/or counseling are beneficial. It won't be the first time the doctor has encountered a patient who smokes dope or takes drugs, and sadly it won't be the last. If your own doctor makes you too uncomfortable, try calling a clinic or "hot line." They will be able to put you in touch with someone who specializes in drugs.

Feeling guilty and spending hours worrying about having had a few drinks at the last cookout, smoking a pack of cigarettes a day, or indulging in an occasional joint will probably have a more deleterious effect than the act itself. It is better to say, "I did something I shouldn't have. I'll try not to do it again."

A pregnant woman can choose what goes into her body. The baby can't. Before drinking quantities of soda pop, smoking cigarettes, or having a joint, ask yourself, "Am I willing to take a chance with the health and well-being of my baby?"

DIET

The importance of a good diet during pregnancy is universally accepted. For the cesarean mother, it is even more important. The physical stress of the cesarean delivery (from surgery, anesthesia, and medications) will deplete vitamins and minerals excessively, although temporarily. After the baby is born, the mother's body will be extremely taxed in caring for her newborn and coping with the regular household chores.

This book does not attempt to explore diet and nutrition in depth, because there are numerous books that thoroughly cover the subject of nutrition. Agricultural extension agencies and the U.S. Government Printing Office are other excellent sources of inexpensive, informative material on diet and food preparation.

We all know what is proper nutritionally; but what we *should* be eating does not always coincide with what we actually put into our bodies. A general rule to follow is to include foods from each food group daily (protein, vegetables, fruits, and grains) and to eat foods as close to the way nature made them as possible (and palatable). Most obstetricians routinely prescribe prenatal vitamins as a supplement and safeguard. It is a good idea to take them faithfully even if your diet is excellent. Some vitamins, such as vitamin C, are rapidly depleted and must be replenished daily. If you prefer organic or natural vitamins to the ones prescribed by your doctor, ask for a sample of the prescribed brand (provided to the doctor free by the manufacturer). Coordinate the dosage of vitamins and minerals in the prescription tablets to organic vitamin supplements. You will probably have to take more than one capsule, but the effort is worthwhile because organic vitamins and minerals are more easily assimilated than chemical preparations.

Remember that the best prenatal diets do not necessarily include extra calories (unless you are underweight) but do include meaningful calories. Adhere to the dictum, "Making each calorie count is more important than counting each calorie." Proper diet during pregnancy is essential to feeling good during pregnancy, nourishing your unborn baby, more quickly recovering from the rigors of labor and delivery, and caring for a newborn. In order to meet your body's and your baby's needs during pregnancy and lactation, extra fluids are necessary. Water has no calories and quenches thirst while providing additional fluid intake. Pure fruit juices are preferable to drinks that are primarily sugar and water. Vegetarian mothers-to-be should also make certain that they are obtaining sufficient quantities of protein daily. This may require the addition of fish or chicken to the vegetarian diet. Protein is essential in that it builds and maintains all tissues, supplies energy, and is a main source of enzymes, hormones, and body fluids.

Breakfast is the most important meal of the day. Your body has been without food for many hours and needs to be nourished. If morning sickness occurs in early pregnancy, it's okay to delay breakfast. Eat as soon as you feel able to. If you skip breakfast, you'll be tired and dragged out, and you may even become dizzy. To help overcome queasiness, eat soda crackers before getting up.

Bake your own bread if you have the time and inclination. Use whole-wheat flour or add soy granules, nonfat dry milk, or wheat germ to give your baked goods (bread, muffins, rolls, cakes, or cookies) additional nutritive value. If you must rely on store-bought bread, think about buying oatmeal, whole-wheat, or whole-grain varieties. Most soft commercial white breads have had nutrients and fiber removed in processing.

Keep your consumption of sugar to a minimum. Sugar is caloric and non-nutritive, and it is not easily assimilated. For sweeteners, use honey, maple syrup, or molasses as much as possible in coffee and tea and on toast. Since coffee, tea and cola contain caffeine, they, too, should be eliminated or reduced in quantity.

To avoid constipation and hemorrhoids (a frequent malady during pregnancy), eat lots of fiber foods, fresh vegetables, fruits, and foods rich in vitamin B complex (yeast, liver, whole grain cereals).

For nibbles and snacks, instead of the usual junk foods, try the following nutritious and delicious ideas suggested by pregnant women. You may find them a welcome variation from your usual diet.

raisins

unsalted nuts

yogurt (make your own flavors at a lower price than the individual containers by purchasing a quart of plain, unflavored yogurt; then add honey, wheat germ, jam, fresh fruit, etc.)

fresh fruit

raw vegetables with or without a dip (eating lots of raw vegetables and fruit will help prevent constipation)

cottage cheese

cheese (the natural varieties such as cheddar or swiss, rather than the processed type such as Velveeta) with or without whole-wheat or whole-grain crackers

oatmeal bread with honey

a peanut butter and honey sandwich

super shakes (milk blended with ice cream and/or bananas and/or a raw egg and/or chocolate and/or vanilla extract and/or strawberries —quick, light, and easy to digest)

cereal and milk and fruit (toasted wheat germ, honey, and fruit are great!)

predigested liquid protein (available at health food stores and a quick pick-me-up)

shrimp cocktail

an avocado and sprout sandwich

chef's salad (an anything-goes combination, such as lettuce, shredded cabbage, carrots, grated cheese, sliced or diced leftover meat, raisins, sunflower seeds, raw or cooked and chilled cauliflower or broccoli, grated or sliced zucchini or summer squash, sprouts, croutons, avocado slices, artichoke hearts, boiled eggs, etc.)

Eating well, obtaining adequate rest, exercising, and abstaining from drugs is essential to your baby's growth and development and to supplying yourself with the resources needed to keep fit and well. If you have maintained an adequate diet during pregnancy, when the time comes for you to have your baby your body will have a storehouse of vitamins and minerals on which to draw. If you feel physically well during pregnancy, you will be able to cope more effectively with caring for the baby and seeing yourself through the postpartum period. Good nutrition is an insurance policy for both the unborn baby and the mother.

Your diet should not undergo a drastic change during pregnancy (unless your obstetrician has special reasons for insisting that you stick to a prescribed diet), although pregnancy is often a good time to gradually introduce new foods to yourself and your family. And don't be a martyr *all* the time. Treat yourself and your family to occasional "splurges." We all need rewards sometimes.

Your pregnant body will place extra demands upon you. Prenatal vitamins and minerals will supplement your diet, but they should not be relied on as replacements for any foods—especially raw fruits and vegetables. Feeling well during pregnancy will make the potential stress of an operative delivery less taxing and will probably decrease the amount of time it takes you to recover fully. The demands of pregnancy, surgery, childbirth, and child care are great. All pregnant women, and especially cesarean mothers, are well advised to provide themselves with adequate resources to cope happily and healthily.

EXERCISE

Exercise, combined with a good diet, is the best insurance policy a pregnant woman can have. Like a health plan or life insurance, it pays regular dividends from the very first day; and you can "borrow" against it when you need it during pregnancy, childbirth, and later when you are recuperating.

Why should a woman who is to deliver by cesarean need any exercise? After all, she probably won't have to prepare herself for the rigors of labor, right? True, labor may usually be forestalled in mandatory cesareans by scheduling the delivery in advance of the due date. Getting into or staying in shape during pregnancy is important to speed up the recovery process. If you have your baby in a state of fitness (fitness does not mean bulging muscles), you will be better able to care for yourself and your baby. Your figure will return more quickly, and getting back into shape soon after delivery will be good for your soul as well as your body.

The easiest, cheapest, and most convenient form of exercise during pregnancy is walking. The fresh air is good for you and your baby. Walking will make the strain of carrying around almost twenty extra pounds easier. It also promotes relaxation and muscle tone. If you are in shape during pregnancy, the delivery may go easier for you, and it will make those first few days and weeks after the baby is born more comfortable.

Unless you were a physical fitness aficionada before pregnancy, the thought of daily exercise at this time may be less than welcome. You may feel too tired, too big, too ... But as an expectant mother, you have one really positive thing going for you: motivation. Most pregnant women are highly motivated to ensure the best possible start for their babies. This includes diet, prenatal visits, vitamins, and exercise.

No exercise program should begin with a vigorous workout one day and sore muscles the next. You won't want to continue. Before beginning any exercise program, check with your doctor. Always begin slowly and build up.

Any exercise regularly undertaken before pregnancy can usually be continued during pregnancy. If you swam, rode horseback, or played tennis daily, you will probably be allowed to continue—but check with your doctor first. A few sports are prohibited and dangerous during pregnancy, including scuba diving, skydiving, and water-skiing.

Whatever exercise you do, pursue it on a regular basis. Try to make it interesting and enjoyable. Yoga is one example of an exercise that combines discipline of the mind with that of the body. It is also a superior form of relaxation, and you will find the ability to relax helpful when the time comes for prenatal tests, having your baby, and coping with a cesarean recovery and a new baby at the same time. If you are interested in yoga, I recommend *Yoga for New Parents* by Ferris Urbanowski. Also recommended are the exercise books by Jane Fonda and Elizabeth Noble.

RELAXATION BREATHING TECHNIQUES

Most prepared childbirth programs ready couples for labor and delivery by means of relaxation breathing techniques. There are different techniques with various names (Lamaze, Kitzinger, Bing, etc.), but the purpose of each one is to train the mind through control and concentration to alleviate the discomforts of labor. Why then do cesarean mothers need these skills?

Braxton Hicks Contractions. During pregnancy the cesarean mother experiences these testing contractions, which ready the uterus for labor. (For more information about Braxton Hicks contractions, see pages 94–95.)

Pelvic Examinations. Internal examinations do not usually hurt, but they can be embarrassing, uncomfortable, or tension producing. Relaxation breathing techniques will be helpful whenever you have to have an internal examination.

Delivery. During delivery it is still possible to feel minor sensation even with a spinal or epidural anesthetic. These sensations may feel like pressure, pulling, or tugging. (For more information, see Chapter 8.) These sensations do not mean that the anesthesia has failed to work, but you will want to know how to relax to reduce discomfort.

Postpartum Contractions. Within a very short time after the baby has been born, your uterus will start to contract to its normal nonpregnant size. These postpartum uterine contractions are similar to labor contractions. Relaxation breathing will help you to cope.

Postpartum Discomfort. Uncomfortable feelings after delivery range from mild to acute. Formerly effortless movements, such as turning, sitting, walking, sneezing, and coughing, may be painful for a few days. Controlled, relaxed breathing will help you to cope more comfortably and effectively.

Tests of Fetal Maturity and Well-Being. These tests are being used more frequently today and may be stress-producing situations. Relaxation breathing will be helpful if your doctor orders an amniocentesis or stress test (see page 80).

Most Westerners think of breathing techniques as a sort of Oriental mumbo-jumbo. There is no mumbo-jumbo involved, no arcane mysticism. If need be, a nurse can teach you some of the more salient points of relaxation breathing techniques in just a few minutes. But why wait until you are experiencing extreme anxiety or discomfort before availing yourself of these methods? Relaxation breathing is a skill that can be acquired in just a few minutes (though practice is helpful), and it is one that will stand you in good stead for the rest of your life. Even when your childbearing years are over, there will still be times when you become tense. Within the context of pregnancy and childbirth, relaxation breathing techniques are a tool, a valuable resource on which to draw to "stay on top" of tension or discomfort.

Controlled Relaxation Breathing. This is the easiest technique, and it can be done at any time, anywhere, and does not require special equipment or preparation.

Take in a deep breath and then let out all the air. (This breath is called a welcoming breath.) This will provide you with additional oxygen. Then breathe in slowly through your nose to the count of three. On three, begin to let the air out through pursed lips, again to the count of three. Do this several times, as necessary. To end the exercise, take in another deep breath (a relaxation or parting breath), and let it out. You might want to time yourself, or have a partner time you. Use 30, 60, and 90 seconds as intervals of time in which to practice.

Dissociative Breathing and Touch Relaxation. When you become tense emotionally, the muscles in your body become tense, too. Conversely, if part of your body becomes tense, or is subjected to an unwelcome pain stimulus, your mind will tense up. You will want to know how to control your mind to relax your body. In other words, you will want to block out the pain stimuli so that they are unable to maintain control over your thought processes.

To practice dissociative breathing techniques and touch relaxation, it is better to have a partner who can keep a close check on you and help you be aware of parts of your body that are still tense.

Lie on your side on a bed, mat, or floor, with several layers of blanket under you. Place pillows under your head and between your knees, which should be flexed. It is better to practice on your left side to keep the full weight of the baby off the vena cava (see page 30). The object of this practice is to achieve a deep sense of relaxation for both your muscles and your mind.

Determine if you feel more comfortable with your eyes open or closed by practicing both ways. If your eyes are open, concentrate on a shape. Don't glare at the shape—that will only increase the tension. Simply use it for a focal area. (An excellent focal area is the face of your mate or coach. Posters, paintings, and mobiles also make good focal areas.)

Take a deep welcoming breath in and let it out. Then, as you breathe in slowly through your nose and out through pursed lips, imagine that your body is melting, that it has become as limp as a rag doll or a plate of overcooked spaghetti. When you begin to practice, it may be necessary to give messages to all the muscles to relax. Start at your toes: tell them to relax. Work your way up so that every part of your body becomes soft and relaxed. Continue to breathe in slowly through your nose, then let the breath out through your mouth (which will probably be slack if you are comfortable and relaxing well). While you are doing this controlled, gentle breathing, your coach should be able to lift any part of you and feel its entire and total weight. You offer no resistance. You cannot help to pick up or put down the arm or leg your coach is supporting. When the time interval (clocked by your coach) is over, your coach will release your arm or leg. Take a deep parting breath in and let it out. Practice your breathing exercises several times a day. When the session is over, remember that you should *not* go suddenly from a position flat on the floor to a full sit or stand. If you do, you may become dizzy. As Sheila Kitzinger, the noted British childbirth educator, advises, whenever you get up after lying down, pretend that you are Cleopatra rising slowly and elegantly from her barge. Cleopatra would not have jumped up like a rabbit. You shouldn't either. Always, always turn on your side, rest there until you want to stand, and use your hands to help lift your body. If you try to accomplish a straight sit-up when getting out of bed or finishing your relaxation breathing practice session, you'll find the strain on your abdominal muscles great.

To help determine what you look like when you are relaxed, your coach should observe you while you are sound asleep. If your coach is your mate, he will know which parts of your body are most likely to be more tense than others. Some people squint their eyes, others tighten the muscles in their forehead or back, some grit their teeth or clench their jaws or fist. After a few practice sessions, your coach should be able to pinch you (hard!) on any part of your body. If you have become well versed in dissociative breathing techniques, you will be aware of the pressure, but not the pain.

If your background includes yoga, meditation, or any similar discipline, relaxation will be almost second nature to you. The important thing is to devise a means of transcending the physical plane in a manner that works well for you. You may want to focus on a shape, silently chant a word or phrase, or envision a lovely scene.

Proficiency in relaxation and controlled breathing techniques is every bit as helpful to the cesarean mother as it is to any other expectant mother. If you spend only five or ten minutes a day practicing (with an occasional day off as a sort of positive stroke to the ego) you will have sufficient time to learn how to control your mind and body in order to conquer discomfort and tension.

A note regarding all special breathing techniques designed for pregnancy, labor and delivery. Almost every one has at one time or another been criticized for being ineffective, counterproductive, too rigid and/or of little or questionable value. In fact, some contemporary childbirth advocates contend that no laboring woman needs to be taught how to breathe, that doing what comes naturally is preferable to a preordained breathing pattern. What is imperative is that you try to remain in control and be as relaxed as possible. Anxiety, muscle tension, panic and fear reduce the flow of oxygen to both mother and baby and may inhibit labor and delivery. At some point, many women lose control, at least for a few minutes. They yell, swear, beseech the staff, beg God, and curse those around them, particularly the baby's father. There comes a time during each woman's labor when she feels she cannot go on and says so in no uncertain terms. That this is a common reaction and not a unique phenomenon does not make it any easier when you are the woman in labor. Breathing conditioning and relaxation techniques are crutches to help see you through these rough times.

TELLING THE CHILDREN

Most children assume that babies come out of the mother's tummy—after all, that's where they grow. Thus, explaining the cesarean delivery to a child can sometimes be easier than explaining a vaginal delivery. However, you should explain to children that there are two ways of having a baby. How much you tell them, and when, will depend on your children's ages and how comfortable you feel with the subject.

Pregnancy is a good time to introduce the subject of how babies are made. Little children will be fascinated to feel the baby kick. It makes the new baby seem more real to them and in the long run will probably help to reduce the amount of sibling jealousy.

It is also important to explain to children that you will need to spend a few days in the hospital when the baby is born. It's rather an unpleasant surprise for children not to know that Mommy will be leaving for a few days and then have her return home with an "intruder" in her arms.

Mothers are usually more concerned about hospitalization than their children are. As long as your children are happy with the person who takes care of them and have special activities planned, your absence will probably have little negative effect. Crying and being sad that you have to go away for a few days is normal. Little children's sense of time is not well developed and they probably won't be as aware of how long you are gone as you are. In fact, many a mother has returned home to find her older children paying more attention to the television or a toy than to her!

EMOTIONAL STRESS:
THE FEAR FACTOR

These comments were made by parents who had no preparation to help them cope with an emergency cesarean delivery. All echo the need for education and support.

"I'm just not ready to be a mother."

"The responsibilities of fatherhood are overwhelming. Why are we having a baby now?"

"I shouldn't have been in such a hurry to have a baby. I had a career I really liked."

"Maybe we should have waited longer ... paid off the house ... traveled more ... become more secure financially."

"Bill and I really wanted this baby. We planned to have it. It wasn't an accident. We waited until we thought we were ready. Now I don't know. Some days I feel trapped. I'm scared. How are we going to be able to cope?"

"I'm afraid my baby will be deformed or retarded."

"I'm afraid the strain of having another baby will destroy our relationship. It's so fragile now. Herb wasn't much help after the first one. How's he going to react this time?"

These feelings may be voiced by *any* parent and are probably no more or less acute in cesarean pregnancies. But there can be an additional stress with a cesarean. Here are some reactions from cesarean parents-to-be:

"I'm afraid to have another section. The first one was awful. I was in labor for what seemed like years before I had the section. It hurt so much afterward, too. It took me six months before I felt like a real human being again. I didn't even know that the baby had been born until the next day. When I woke up, I thought I was still in labor. I'm so afraid to go through that again. But now it's too late. For me it's the only way I can have a baby."

"I'm happy to be pregnant again. It took so long to conceive the first baby. Then I had two miscarriages before this pregnancy. I really do want this baby. But I hate the thought of getting anesthesia and being all cut up again."

"I thought I was going to die. They kept giving me something to bring on contractions and then they'd zonk me out with something else. I was so lonely and confused by that time. When they said they were going to do a cesarean, I welcomed the announcement. I think what bothered me more than anything was that there were a bunch of interns around my bed. They kept talking about me as though I was a cadaver. They said things to each other like, 'Her pulse is failing.' and 'I can't get the baby's heartbeat.' There were a lot of other women in that big room and they were all moaning, 'Help me, help me, please. Won't somebody help me, I'm dying.' This was my first baby so I assumed they knew more than I did. If they were dying, I figured I might be, too. And when the interns said they couldn't get the baby's heartbeat, it meant my baby was dead. The final, ultimate insult was to hear one of them say, 'The full moon sure brought out a bunch of weirdos.' So there I was, a dying weirdo with a dead baby. My son was born healthy, but it wasn't thanks to the tender loving care I got."

"I know I should feel grateful. I would have died, and the baby, too, if I had lived fifty or a hundred years ago. But the

section was so unplanned. We didn't want to be pulled away from each other when the going got tough. The doctor made Jerry leave, and I wanted him to stay. He left, but not willingly. At the hospital where I'm going fathers are not allowed to be with their wives at all for a section. It's so sad, really. This is our last baby. We wanted to share the first one's birth, and now we won't even be able to be together for this one. I wish there was something we could do."

"My mother had two cesareans. She said she almost died each time. She was so afraid she'd get pregnant again that she wouldn't let my father touch her. But that was many years ago. More than anything in the world, I wanted to avoid having a section. I was floored when the doctor said the baby was breech and that I might have to have a cesarean. It wasn't as bad as I thought it would be, but it wasn't very nice. The doctor tried to give me a spinal and it didn't work so I got put out. I hated it. I couldn't believe how much pain there was afterward. I'm afraid. I don't want to have to go through the pain again. Other women say it isn't so awful to have a cesarean . . . but I don't know . . . it sure hurt like hell."

"Doctors charge an extra fee for doing a section. It's such a rip-off. It probably takes them less time, especially with a repeat 'cause they can schedule when they have to come in. It takes only an hour. Sometimes they have to spend hours and hours waiting in the hospital while a woman's in labor. They shouldn't charge extra for doing a cesarean—they should charge less. Cesarean parents have to pay extra for everything. It's a form of discrimination, and I don't like it. Besides, we can't afford to have a baby. I'm really worried about all those bills. I got pregnant and then my husband got laid off so we don't have any insurance. You've gotta be either extra-rich or extra-poor in order to get medical care. If you're in the middle like us, you pay through the nose."

"I had my appendix out a few years ago. It almost burst right before Thanksgiving dinner. I wasn't scared then. I was in too much pain, and it was the first time anyone had paid me that much attention. I was just glad to get it over with. Two years ago I had an emergency c-sec. I was scared to death. Appendix is one thing, but a baby, why, that's something else. I was afraid I would die. I was afraid the doctor would cut the baby by accident. I was afraid my guts would spill out onto the floor the first time I got out of bed. I was afraid to hold the baby. I was afraid I wouldn't be a good mother. I was afraid to take the baby home. I felt lousy. It was so hard, taking care of a baby and getting over the operation. When I had my appendix out, I could go home and rest and recuperate. It was the same kind of thing—the operation, that is. I mean, it's done almost the same way. But my appendix wasn't handed to me wrapped in a blanket for feedings at 2 A.M."

"What was the best part? Geeze, there wasn't any good part. It was all pretty bad. I mean, aside from having a beautiful baby and all. You know, I think the doctor really genuinely thinks he did a good job. I mean, he did spend a lot of time with me when I went to his office. But he never really answered my questions. He just sort of said, 'Well, it's okay. Just leave everything to me.' When I was in the hospital, the nurses made me feel like I was bothering them when I called for help. I tried not to think about myself too much, and concentrated on the baby. But it hurt a lot. I didn't want my husband to think I wasn't happy to have the baby. I was. But I don't want to go through that again. Not alone, not without someone to understand how I felt, how much help I needed. I hate being dependent on anyone. But I really had to lean on everyone—the nurses, my husband, and my mother, who came to help after the baby was born."

"None of my friends had sections. They made me feel like a weirdo for not being able to do it 'their' way, the 'right' way. After a while, I didn't even want to see them again. They were so condescending. They did everything within a week after the baby was born. I was still in the hospital. Then when I got home, I felt like a zombie. Oh, they complained about their long labors and their episiotomies and their hemorrhoids. But I had a long, hard labor, too, and a huge stomach cut and hemorrhoids."

"It's too bad there isn't any information for cesareans. It would have made things a lot easier on us if we could have found out about it before it happened."

"I didn't know what to expect, and when it was all over, I didn't know what had happened, only that it did happen. I wish I knew what happened, and why, and how my baby was born. I felt like we were functioning in a vacuum. I get scared when I don't know what to expect. It's a lot better—and easier to deal with—if you know what's going to happen, and how it's going to feel. I want the next baby to be born while I'm awake. It's kind of like the difference between giving birth under a bushel basket and having a baby out in the open."

"My mother told me never to get pregnant again after I had my first cesarean. When I did, she told me I'd better take out a life insurance policy on myself 'cause I'd never make it off the operating table alive."

"I know this isn't true only of cesarean mothers, but I felt like a pawn in a chess game. I chose to go to a certain doctor because I heard he was real good. But when I got to my first visit, I was told, not asked, that I would see a different one of the three doctors each time. Well, I know I shouldn't say this but . . . I really took an instant disliking to one of them. The other one was okay. My face must have dropped down to the floor each time someone other than 'my' doctor came into the room—the first time especially. I think there's something very important about establishing a good relationship with your doctor. It can be a father-daughter relationship, or a brother-sister thing, or a friend-to-friend kind of thing. I resented the fact that I was paying for the services of one doctor, and had to settle for the other ones. It was my money, and I felt terrible but I was too intimidated to speak up. I tried it once, with the receptionist, but all she said was, 'That's just the way we do things here. It's better for you to see all the doctors. You can't *do it your way.' I dropped the subject after that. It was too much trouble to pursue it, and I didn't want to hurt the other doctors' feelings. It was just my rotten luck to get the one I liked least to do the cesarean. I felt disappointed. I think I wouldn't have minded so much if I'd gotten the doctor I liked best."*

"The only thing I could find out about cesarean sections was that there wasn't any information. So I asked around. All I heard were scare stories. So I stopped asking."

"Hal and I bought every book on childbirth we could find. I'd come back from the library with so many books I could hardly hold them all. We read every word. Then I had a surprise cesarean. So I went back to those books and looked up the word. You know what? Some of them didn't even mention it! And in others, there was so little as to be almost useless. Usually it didn't even say anything about cesareans, other than that it was an operation. What killed me were the ones that said you could avoid having a section if you minded your p's and q's. Hey, I did that! I was really looking forward to having my first baby. And I was religious about practicing and exercising. I was better about doing my exercises and breathing than anyone else in our class! So I felt like a failure and an ignorant fool. What concerns me is that I want to make the next birth better. I want it to be a good thing, not only for me but for my baby and my husband. He felt so cheated. I don't want it to be the horror show it was before, although mine wasn't as bad as some of the women I've talked to. But I am very much afraid. I know I shouldn't be, but I know that anesthesia can be dangerous. . . . I know that the baby can be born with breathing problems like the Kennedy baby. . . . I know that I could get a terrible infection . . . and I know that I'm being too much of a worrywart. My head tells me that everything will be all right. But my heart says, 'Look out, with your luck, anything that could go wrong will.'"

The "fear factor" of a cesarean birth can involve many things including:

  1. The responsibilities of parenthood.
  2. The loss of income if the mother has been

working, coupled with the extra cost of a cesarean delivery and the financial strain of supporting another child.

3. Fear that the baby will be less than perfect, that she or he will be damaged or defective.

4. Guilt that negative emotions crop up at a time in one's life when everything is *supposed* to be beautiful and perfect, when the anticipation of a new baby is *supposed* to bring joy, not resentment.

5. The fears of *any* person about to undergo any type of surgery. These fears are accented in the case of cesarean parents, for the family will be simultaneously involved in both childbirth *and* surgery.

6. The almost total lack of solid, helpful information. Couples have often had to rely on myths, misinformation, and old wives' tales. The experiences of other cesarean mothers, who may relate tales of horror, however true or false these impressions may be, undermine much of the confidence pregnant cesarean couples have developed on their own.

7. Memory of previous experiences that may have been fraught with pain and/or psychological and physical stress.

8. Condescension by one's peers who may see the cesarean mother as a failure. This attitude, combined with the fact that the mother may already feel inadequate, is sufficient to create numerous problems.

9. Possible lack of rapport between doctor and client as a result of personality conflict, the lack of alternative doctors and/or hospitals (as is the case in areas where the population is not dense enough to give expectant couples a choice), specialization (a different doctor is called in to treat various members of each family, and different medical conditions for each member), or the growing number of team practices that do not take into account the fact that the woman may not wish to be cared for by all members of the group but prefers one doctor to the others.

10. The lack of prenatal classes and support groups for expectant cesarean parents in many areas of the country.

11. The lack of postpartum help and support for the

cesarean mother both in the hospital and after returning home.

12. The fear that you may fail if you attempt to deliver vaginally after one or more previous cesareans. Should your VBAC not succeed, you may have to contend with the idea that you failed again. However, if you did everything in your power to avoid a cesarean, you should take pride in the fact that you tried.

Women who deliver vaginally and who have had very negative birth experiences do not relish the thought of going through "that" again, and the prospect of an elective or repeat cesarean may carry with it the same impact as knowing almost a full year in advance that you have an appointment with a particularly sadistic dentist. The anticipation of childbirth-cum-surgery or surgery-cum-childbirth, as the case may be, is the major "fear factor" in cesarean pregnancies *unless* cesarean parents are given the skills needed to help themselves achieve better birthing experiences.

How many women sail through a cesarean delivery with nary a negative thought and without a moment's pain? Surely there are some who do not find the experience the least bit difficult, trying, or disconcerting. Others may be so happy to have a baby after years of infertility that the result more than justifies the means. However, women who find the experience easy and completely without discomfort or tension are probably in the minority.

The keys to alleviating the additional psychological stress of a cesarean delivery are education and empathy. That tired old phrase, "We have nothing to fear but fear itself" has special meaning for cesarean couples. Knowing what to expect and how to cope is the best preparation and the only defense against fear.

Enlightenment follows education. As information about cesarean childbirth and vaginal birth after cesarean (VBAC) becomes more widely available, traditional attitudes will cesarean parents are developing a new, raised consciousness,

Recipe

Take: two parents-to-be who may experience a temporary panic as they contemplate the responsibilities of parenthood and their unpreparedness for taking care of a newborn.

Add: a dash of fear that the baby may be born less than perfect.

Fold in: the parents' guilt that they are having negative thoughts in the first place.

Combine: the ordinary trepidations of anyone about to have surgery.

Take away: books, films, and slides concerning this alternative birthing method.

Remove: classes in prepared childbirth designed to meet the special needs of these parents (because no one thought they were needed).

Beat in: two lumps of confusion on behalf of maternity personnel who are not quite certain about their roles in caring for a patient who is both postpartum and postsurgical.

Throw in: anxiety, tension, myths, and misinformation— and the often harrowing experiences of others.

Separate: parents just when they need each other's love and support most.

Optional: one or more previous cesarean deliveries.

Wheel: your mixture into an operating room and keep there for about one hour, or until done.

Yield: one cesarean section, hopefully one healthy baby, and two traumatized parents.

change. Many cesarean parents are developing a new, raised consciousness, which will extend from these parents to doctors, nurses, hospital administrators, childbirth educators, friends, family, and everyone with whom cesarean parents come into contact. Where previously the cesarean mother may have been neither fish nor fowl (she was not just a postsurgical patient, nor was she *only* a regular postpartum maternity patient) and could not therefore be neatly categorized, she will now benefit from a new status that takes into account her very special physical and emotional needs. Like all mothers, she is entitled to the best possible care, including support for a safe, positive birth experience when a cesarean is inevitable, and backup for her desires to go into labor spontaneously and attempt vaginal delivery whenever possible.

Empathy is needed from everyone who comes into contact with cesarean parents, be it on a friendship or professional basis. Friends can learn to respect the cesarean mother rather than look down on her. Families need no longer feel sorry for her. Childbirth educators will no longer see these couples as oddities or failures who didn't follow their advice, instruction, and rules. Cesarean parents do not want to be smothered in sympathy or coldly rejected. But they *do* need empathy, education, support, encouragement, and a new understanding of their special needs.

Anyone who has ever had major surgery can remember the difficulties involved. Anyone who has ever had a baby knows what child care entails. We should ask, "What must it feel like to have a baby *and* an operation?" "Should we expect cesarean women to automatically, magically transform themselves into 'good' and caring mothers at a time when their own physical limitations make them potentially (and very understandably) egocentric?" Any parent who has had a baby by cesarean knows the answers to these questions. As one nurse said, "I thought cesarean mothers were a big pain in the neck. They were always calling the station for help. Then I got pregnant and had to have a c-section. Boy, did my attitude change in a hurry!"

It is not necessary for a childbirth instructor to have had a cesarean to teach cesarean couples—but it helps. Male doctors, however well-intentioned, cannot know how their clients feel, but they *can* sympathize. Regarding their patients as pregnant uteri that must be incised may help doctors in their job of objectively making decisions, but it does not encourage their understanding of their clients as people. The nurse or doctor who has never had a baby, or who had a vaginal delivery, or who delivered so many years ago that there were few differences between how mothers were treated regardless of the method of delivery can still be a tremendous help to the cesarean family.

Health care professionals can begin to reassess their attitudes. They could start by imagining how they would feel if a doctor or nurse walked into their rooms and said (as some doctors and nurses now say), "Stop blubbering. Stop bemoaning your fate. You had a baby. It's healthy. Why are you so upset? It's nothing. You'll get over it." The nurse who breezes into the room of a newly delivered cesarean mother, leaves the baby's crib ten feet away from the mother's bed, and then zips out almost as quickly as she came in might stop a minute to picture how she would feel if she were the mother in that bed. Most nurses are *not* callous or unconcerned. The problem has often been that some nurses simply have never given much thought to the plight of the cesarean mother who is initially quite physically handicapped, who may feel helpless, alone, frightened, or uncomfortable, and who is completely unable to get out of bed without assistance, much less get the baby back into bed with her. Cesarean fathers who find themselves short on understanding might also try to put themselves in their wives' situation. How would they feel being uncomfortable physically and almost totally dependent on others for help?

In-service training programs are now being offered in a number of hospitals to increase the level of understanding with regard to present systems of care for cesarean families. Newspapers and magazines are catching on to the fact that articles about cesarean sections and VBACs are timely and of interest to readers. Childbirth education associations are to be credited with improving the care and handling of vaginal deliveries. Now, fortunately, many of them are devoting some effort to taking the cesarean out of the dark ages and enlightening families about VBACs.

"I just never thought about it that way" is a remark frequently made by health care professionals, childbirth educators, editors, and noncesarean parents. Because the majority of cesarean deliveries performed today are *technically* perfect, the very false assumption has been that there is no need to concern oneself with the *emotional* well-being of cesarean couples. Unless cesarean couples speak up and speak out, it is possible for hundreds of poor-quality (from the psychological aspect) cesarean deliveries to take place without anyone in the hospital giving the procedure, or the people who have experienced it, more than passing thought. The doctor may admire the precision of the incision, the neatness of the scar. The anesthesiologist may wonder at the ease with which the anesthesia was administered. Nurses may congratulate themselves on their efficiency. And the parents may be totally drained by the experience. They take their babies home from the hospital thinking that they are glad to be out of there, and wondering why they don't feel more grateful for such expert care.

It is difficult, if not impossible, for many people to express their concerns. If previous cesarean deliveries were harrowing and left bitter impressions, the results can sometimes be measured by the degree of withdrawal, fright, hostility, or displaced anger experienced. Often, cesarean parents simply "grin and bear it," "keep a stiff upper lip," and adhere to all the other cliches about keeping one's problems to oneself. If cesarean parents do not talk about how they feel, no one is going to know how to help them. Organizations for cesarean and VBAC parents are being formed in many areas throughout the country. They are excellent sources of information and support. Together parents will be able to talk about their experiences with others who can truly understand. Together they will be able to work through and finalize the experience, and move on to more positive attitudes. Together they will share tips on how to cope with situations and bring about change. Together they can achieve better-quality health care for themselves and for future cesarean and VBAC parents as well.

Doctors, hospital administrators, childbirth educators, and maternity nurses should be approached with determination about the goals, complaints, questions, and comments of cesarean parents. If they are doing their jobs well in their own eyes, suggestions for change may meet with initial resistance. Give them time. You may have been thinking about the subject for weeks or months, but your suggestions are new to *them*. Be patient and persistent. Understanding cannot grow in a climate of hostility or aggression. But it will come with time, persistence, and patience.

There may not be enough time to achieve all your goals while you are pregnant. But your efforts will not be in vain, for they will help others. Your enthusiasm will be passed on to other parents, to your children, to family, friends, and health care professionals.

Cesarean mothers do not have to live in fear of the impending delivery. With the sharing of efforts and the cooperation of others, they can look forward to a birthing experience that is positive, joyous, and comfortable. As understanding grows, tension and fear will decrease. There should be *no* stigma associated with having a cesarean delivery. It can and should be regarded as an experience to be met with confidence and joy.

AFTER DELIVERY

If the trauma of the birth has left scars on a woman's psyche, they may not fade as quickly as the one on her abdomen, and it may be necessary for her to seek professional counseling. Usually, though, psychological distance and a lapse of time between the mother and her birth experience will help put negative feelings in perspective. Temporary feelings of anger, resentment, failure, frustration, guilt and/or depression are not unusual.

Unfortunately, many cesarean birth experiences are still harrowing and emotionally stressful. It is also true that a few cesarean mothers use their birth experiences as scapegoats for earlier, unrelated problems, such as marital troubles or deep-seated chronic depression. A host of unrelated physical ailments, such as lack of sexual arousal and interest, weight gain, or headaches may also be blamed on the cesarean delivery.

In the first few months after delivery, the lack of sexual desire may cause the mother to think that she has become frigid. It is difficult—if not impossible—to feel amorous when one has been deprived of a full night's sleep for weeks and the house has fallen into rack and ruin because the baby requires so much time. How *do* new parents find the time to make love even if they want to? It can be arranged, but not always easily. (For further discussion, see Chapter 11.) If a woman gains weight, it is not because she had a cesarean but because she is eating too much or not getting enough exercise. Headaches as the result of anesthesia sometimes do occur—but if they do, they will happen within a few days of delivery, not months later.

The cesarean mother may harbor resentment against the baby for being too big or in the wrong position to have been delivered vaginally or for taking up so much of her time after birth; against the doctor for not letting her know what was happening, for allowing her to be in labor so long before making the decision to do a cesarean, or for not allowing her to labor longer to see if she could deliver vaginally; against the nurses for interfering too much or not enough; against the baby's father for making her pregnant in the first place, or for not coaching and supporting her well enough. The list is endless, and not without contradictions.

The new cesarean mother may be angry with herself for accepting or rejecting medication. She may hate her body for being too small, too uncooperative to allow her to have her baby vaginally. She may well think she did something wrong. Birth is supposed to be a normal, natural event, and she could not do it "right." No matter what the indications for her cesarean, no matter what she did or did not do, the fact remains that for the remainder of her life she may have unresolved questions and doubts. "If only I knew then what I know now, I could have avoided a cesarean." "If only I hadn't given up so soon, I might have avoided a cesarean." "If only I had practiced my exercises more." "If I could just do it again, things would be different." "If only . . ."

Frustration may come as the result of listening to friends who have had beautiful, shared vaginal deliveries. They can talk so glowingly of their babies' births—and the cesarean mother may not even be able to remember hers, much less have been able to share it with the baby's father. Her sense of control, her sense of accomplishment, have been taken from her.

Depression immediately after childbirth is a commonly accepted medical condition. No one can, as yet, accurately predict who will get it, why it happens, and what can be done to prevent it. The new cesarean mother may feel like a fool for crying in front of the nurse when she brings in the umpteenth bowl of Jell-O and the mother is so hungry she could eat a six-course dinner for two. Her husband may be bewildered by her behavior when she comes home from the hospital. He cannot understand why she's crying because the baby that they (especially she) wanted and waited for is crying. She may reach the point where she is unable to cope unless she vents her feelings.

No one told the new mother—nor would she have believed—that being a mother can be complicated, time consuming, and almost devoid of creativity and adult companionship. Women pregnant for the first time are notorious for romanticizing what it will be like when the baby comes. They imagine themselves ideal mothers with ideal babies. The reality is that the mother may be crying because she is just as tired, hungry, and in need of love as her baby. The baby's needs have priority. The mother's needs for gratification must be delayed. There are rewards for being a mother, but they may not be apparent for weeks. In the meantime, the only companionship the mother may have during the day is the television and her baby.

Unless the depression is major and long-lasting (in which case the mother will want to see a therapist), it is small consolation to know that she is not alone in her feelings. The best thing she can do is to find other women who are in the same postcesarean, postpartum, new-baby predicament. A local parents' support group or an instructor of prenatal classes should be able to put the mother in touch with other new parents. *Any* new mother, regardless of the method of delivery, is likely to be in the same situation.

Crying is a good release. One should not feel guilty for being resentful, angry, frustrated, or depressed. Guilt will only compound the problem. No one is every admonished for feeling happy, generous, kind, or virtuous, but most of us feel something is intrinsically wrong if we let negative feelings surface. There is something wrong if *all* you are feeling is sad and angry. But you should not be surprised if you are feeling down. You have been through an upheaval that is both physically and emotionally traumatic and exhausting, and you have a right to be on edge, uptight, or blue every now and then.

Postpartum depression may be a commonly accepted medical condition; but there is nothing "routine" about it. It is devastating. Its incidence is so great that it should be considered as a possible diagnosis whenever depressed feelings are very intense or persistent following childbirth.

It is not uncommon to experience *temporary* negative feelings after the baby is born. You may have felt this way even if your baby had been delivered vaginally and all your dreams of the perfect birth had come true. However, there may be a greater sense of failure with a cesarean birth. You didn't fail, but you may think you did. This sense of incompetence may be greater among women whose first cesareans were unplanned. If you are physically exhausted, exhaustion may intensify your feelings of being unable to cope. You may also be jealous of women who have had vaginal births. But it does not help to dwell on depression and to be incapacitated by it. If you hear yourself sounding like a broken record, it's time to change the tune. You may not be able to accomplish it singlehandedly. You will need the help of your husband, family and close friends. Feedback and support from other cesarean parents and concerned professionals can be very beneficial, too. The end product of really working through one's sadness or grief should be a greater ability to accept what happened—even if you still have some negative feelings about it. You may wish to channel your negative feelings into something constructive such as writing letters or articles, helping other cesarean parents, and working for improvements so that parents may benefit from your experiences.

Eventually it should be possible for you to have more positive feelings about your birth experience. These good feelings may come when time has elapsed since the baby's birth. If you have given birth during the winter months, the depression may be greater. As spring comes, you may begin to feel lighter and more agreeable. This will also happen when your baby begins to develop a more manageable routine. Babies are demanding little creatures. The first time your baby smiles at you may just coincide with the end of much of your depression. At last the baby seems to be giving rather than taking.

A cesarean birth is not always easy. But in the words of one mother, "It doesn't have to be so hard. If you know what might happen, you can deal with anything."

TESTS TO DETERMINE FETAL MATURITY AND WELL-BEING

The 1970s brought sophisticated new tests and machines to the field of obstetrics. While these tests may be employed for any pregnancy, they are more common in repeat and elective cesarean deliveries.

Until the introduction of these tests and the surge in VBACs, repeat and elective cesarean births were routinely scheduled to take place about ten days to two weeks before the estimated date of delivery. It takes approximately forty weeks of gestation for the human baby to fully develop and mature. The problem is that babies do not read the books on pregnancy that tell them how long it requires. Some babies take longer than others to ready their systems for life outside the uterus. Prior to the introduction of these new tests, the obstetrician, in scheduling a cesarean delivery, had to rely on time-honored, but less than infallible, considerations such as the mother's estimated date of conception (a date that is likely to be in error), when the mother first felt the baby move (quickening), the height of the fundus (top of the uterus), and signs within the mother's body, such as dilation of the cervix (neck of the uterus), which would indicate that labor was near.

The doctor took these factors into account, along with the

woman's medical history, and tried to schedule an optimal time for both mother and baby so that the baby would be born healthy, full-term, and really able to function independently outside the mother's body. These computations and considerations amounted, in essence, to guesswork. There was no way to gauge surely and accurately what stage of gestation the fetus had reached, nor how well it was progressing in utero. This problem resulted in the traditionally higher incidence of Respiratory Distress Syndrome (RDS) among cesarean-delivered babies.

RDS—a newer and more accurate name for hyaline membrane disease—is a condition wherein the air sacs (alveoli) of the lungs are unable to stay open as they should and collapse after each breath the baby takes. The infant has to work strenuously with each new breath and soon develops numerous physiological and metabolic problems.

Because the incidence of RDS has been higher among cesarean-delivered babies, it became customary to place all cesarean babies in the special care nursery for an observation period of approximately twelve to twenty-four hours, regardless of birth weight, Apgar score (special rating system for newborns, see page 125), or general condition. In special care nurseries, the baby is placed in an isolette (incubator) and the staff watches for possible signs of distress. Special equipment is available should any problems arise.

Tests to determine fetal maturity and well-being are now reducing the risk of RDS and of scheduling a cesarean delivery before the baby is prepared to function independently. The cesarean mother-to-be may have any one or a combination of these tests. She probably will not have all of them. The major consideration is to schedule the birth at a time when the baby is ready. A healthy, full-term infant is the prime concern of both the parents and obstetrician.

Before discussing these antenatal tests, let us not overlook the oldest and best method for determining fetal maturity:

spontaneous labor. As the trend toward subsequent vaginal deliveries grows, and excluding situations in which the mother goes into labor well before the due date, the best way to assess how mature a baby and its lungs are is to wait for the onset of labor. This natural method is also the least intrusive and carries the least risk—and most benefits—to mother and baby. Using a preordained birth date to determine when it is time for a baby to be born is slowly but surely giving way to awaiting the onset of labor. If there is some question regarding fetal well-being and lung maturation, you may undergo one or more of the following tests. You have a right, of course, to refuse to submit to any antenatal tests. The best way to make an intelligent decision is to be well informed. Know what the various tests are and what benefits and risks they carry.

ULTRASOUND OR SONOGRAM

Until fairly recently, x-ray was the only way to determine the size of the fetus. Precautions were taken to diminish the danger of radiation to the baby, but the risk remained. X-rays are now seriously questioned and their use all but abandoned for diagnosing disproportion. It is the potential danger of radiation exposure that gives rise to grave concerns. X-ray is one test I would turn down without hesitation. If x-rays are recommended to determine CPD, remember that the only picture obtained will be one of your baby and your pelvic bones. *The adequacy of a pelvis cannot be determined until you are well into active labor.* The pelvis during labor is different from the pelvis during pregnancy. Nature has built into women's bodies the ability to give birth vaginally even when the pelvis seems "inadequate" or the baby "too large."

Ultrasound utilizes ultrahigh frequency sound waves instead of x-rays to determine the size of the fetus. Although it has not yet been proven if ultrasound carries any risk, it is probably relatively safe provided it is used judiciously. Most hospitals and some doctors' offices today have these machines. An ultrasound test, which may also be called a sonogram, may be able to determine the size of the fetus relative to gestational age, the position of the baby (or babies), where the placenta is located, confirmation of ectopic pregnancy (gestation outside the uterus), fetal breathing, quantity of amniotic fluid, and even fetal muscle tone. The test can also ascertain the baby's gender, although it is by no means infallible. Ultrasound should not be employed just because you want to know what type of clothes to purchase.

Each ultrasound test is costly, but it is painless to the mother and probably harmless to both mother and baby—although it will take another ten to twenty years to determine if, indeed, ultrasound carries risks that are as yet unproven and unknown. When having ultrasound during early pregnancy, the only preparation the mother must make is to have a full bladder, which will show up clearly on the "picture" and can be used as a landmark for interpretation. Having a full bladder at any stage during pregnancy is usually not difficult. In fact, keeping one's bladder empty is often much harder. A full bladder is not required for ultrasound during the last trimester.

State-of-the-art sonogram machines produce more lifelike images than their early prototypes, but it is still difficult for many of us to see as much as the doctors and technicians do. In other words, ultrasonographic pictures do not look like real babies, but it is often possible to pick out the baby's head, arms, legs, etc. Polaroid pictures of the test results are sometimes offered to the parents. Even though you may not be able to interpret them, they are nice keepsakes.

AMNIOCENTESIS

The unborn baby is surrounded by amniotic fluid, which, among other things, washes into and out of the fetal lungs. Amniotic fluid also serves as a protective cushion should the mother experience a blow to her abdomen. As recently as ten years ago, the information contained in amniotic fluid was all but unknown. Now laboratory tests of amniotic fluid can determine such conditions as Rh-sensitized pregnancies, genetic make-up, and fetal lung maturity. Likely candidates for amniocentesis in the last part of the first and early part of the second trimesters of pregnancy are not necessarily the same women who may have an amniotic tap done in the latter part of the third trimester. Amniocentesis (pronounced "am-nee-o-sentee '-sis") is the name for the procedure itself.

Before a sample of the amniotic fluid can be drawn, an ultrasound will be performed to locate the placenta, fetus, and best area from which to draw the sample of amniotic fluid. Probably no test scares expectant parents more than amniocentesis. However, contrary to expectations, a tap is, at most, mildly uncomfortable for the mother.

In order to carry out the procedure, the mother will be given a hospital gown to wear. Before the test begins, make yourself as comfortable and relaxed as possible. I found that having a pillow under my shoulders and another one under my knees made me most comfortable. To alleviate emotional tension or physical discomfort, slow, controlled relaxation breathing is very helpful. (Relaxation breathing techniques are explained starting on page 53.) Bring your mate or a supportive friend with you. Your support person is a good source of comfort and will help you do your controlled relaxation breathing.

Before the tap takes place, various preparations must be made. Your abdomen is first covered with a colorful antiseptic solution, which may feel cool at first. Some doctors inject a local anesthetic to numb the area near where the sample of fluid is to be drawn. Other doctors do not give a local anesthetic, feeling that the discomfort from the injection is as great as the tap itself. (I had three amnioceteses before my daughter, Sarah, was born. It seemed to make no difference in the amount of sensation I could feel whether a local was used or not.)

Once everything has been prepared, the test takes only a few minutes to complete.

As the doctor inserts the cannula (a hollow, slender needle) into the abdomen, you may feel a slight prickling sensation, similar to having a blood sample drawn. Care is taken to ascertain that neither the placenta nor the baby is contacted by the cannula. Also, only a comparatively tiny amount of amniotic fluid is withdrawn.

There are some risks associated with amniocentesis. These risks are small, but they do sometimes occur. One risk is the puncture of the placenta or the fetus. However, if ultrasound is used in conjunction with the tap, the probability of such punctures is minimal. Another risk is miscarriage. In less than 1 percent of all amniotic taps in early pregnancy, miscarriage may take place (this is not true toward the end of pregnancy). In deciding if you should or should not have this procedure done, determine what your priorities are and if the benefits outweigh the risks.

After the amniotic fluid sample has been drawn, a fetal monitor is sometimes used. For parents who have never heard their baby's heartbeat, it is surprising to note that it is normally very fast and sounds like a galloping horse. Variations of 120 to 160 beats per minute are average and normal.

Never insist upon having an amniocentesis simply to determine the sex of your baby. This is irresponsible. Any doctor who would allow expectant parents to indulge in this practice should be avoided. Amniocentesis, and all other forms of obstetrical intervention—including antenatal tests of fetal maturity and well-being—are *serious* and often unnecessary. Too often, the benefits of these interventions accrue only to the financial interests of obstetricians, pharmaceutical companies, diagnostic laboratories, manufacturers of machines, and everyone but the very people they are supposed to help: pregnant parents and unborn babies.

Why an amniotic tap is done, and when, are dependent upon

what type of information is needed. Following are two very important reasons why amniocentesis is peformed.

   Genetic Counseling. Parents-to-be often find themselves in the position of being "at risk" for certain potential problems with their babies. When there is question of chromosome abnormality and/or inherited disease, an amniotic tap may be elected (by parents and/or doctors) in order to determine if, indeed, there is reason to prepare for an abnormality. One of the most common categories of women who will have (or be advised to have) amniocentesis are those thirty-five and over. These women must decide for themselves if they want to go through with the procedure or take their chances. As we know, mothers-to-be in this age group are often well-educated women who established careers for themselves during their twenties and waited until later to have a first or second child. As maternal age advances, the presence of Down's syndrome (mongolism) increases.

A large body of research is currently being conducted and medical innovations are being introduced and refined which mean that genetic tests will soon be able to be undertaken in the first trimester of pregnancy, much earlier than the sixteen to twenty weeks after conception when an amniocentesis is most usually recommended. Because it takes approximately three weeks to grow the fetal cells and study the baby's chromosomes, earlier genetic testing is exceedingly welcomed. As it now stands, a woman must wait until the second trimester before having amniocentesis, then wait almost a month for the results. Chances are more in favor of a normal baby than an abnormal one, and yet, should an abnormal pregnancy be diagnosed, parents who choose to terminate the pregnancy must do so under very adverse conditions: the woman has been pregnant for a relatively long time, and aborting even a severely defective baby after so many months of pregnancy is a difficult choice for most people.

It should be reiterated that having an amniocentesis to make sure there are no chromosomal abnormalities most often results in relief and reassurance. Even though there is some small percentage of error, nonetheless, once you've gotten back good results, you'll be able to go on with your pregnancy with a greater sense of security. You now know that your baby is chromosomally normal. If the test shows abnormality, then you'll be able to either prepare to take on the extra burden of caring for a less-than-perfect child, or make the heart-rending decision to terminate the pregnancy.

Genetic counseling is also advised in other situations. For example, a woman who has had a number of previous spontaneous abortions (miscarriages) may be advised to have amniocentesis to make sure that this time the baby's chromosomes are normal and that there is greater potential to carry a normal baby to term. Families who have had defective babies who died in utero or shortly after birth may want to avail themselves of this procedure to make sure that this will not reoccur. Tay-Sachs carriers and families with a history of congenital abnormalities may also have amniotic taps to determine fetal well-being.

Jonathan Scher, M.D., and Carol Dix in their book *Will My Baby Be Normal? How To Make Sure* offer this encouragement:

> Amniocentesis cannot detect defects of the body structure such as hare lip, cleft palate, clubfoot, congenital heart disease, hypospadias, congenital hip dislocation, or pyloric stenosis. . . . Defects such as these are not caused by chromosomal or genetic defects, but are a result of what we term *multifactorial* reasons. . . . However, [these] structural defects . . . are usually visible on ultrasound, as the newer, more refined machines give such a detailed picture that you can even see the baby's eyelids. And, I firmly believe, we are not far away from

ultrasound so sophisticated that a skilled sonographer will be capable of picking up most structural defects."[1]

Nature is not perfect. Antenatal tests are not perfect, nor are they 100 percent accurate all the time. However, when necessary, they can be a blessing.

Fetal Lung Maturity. Amniocentesis is performed late in pregnancy to evaluate entirely different properties contained within the amniotic fluid, and the results are available within a few hours. Amniocentesis is employed in order to determine the baby's 1/s ratio, that is, the amount of lecithin in the amniotic fluid compared to the amount of sphingomyelin. With a 1/s ratio, it is possible to predict with a fair degree of accuracy how mature the fetal lungs are. Lecithin and sphingomyelin are only two of the properties found in amniotic fluid that relate to fetal lung maturation. Other substances can also be measured, and newer (and perhaps more reliable) tests will soon become widely used in place of or in addition to the one for determining the 1/s ratio. Determining fetal lung maturity for elective and repeat cesareans is one way to prevent delivery of a baby with breathing difficulties. The most common breathing difficulty is Respiratory Distress Syndrome (RDS). The reason for using tests to determine fetal lung maturity is to prevent performing a scheduled cesarean before the baby can breathe on its own outside the uterus.

Determining fetal lung maturity is important in cases where it may be necessary to perform a cesarean well ahead of the due date because of severe maternal illness (e.g., chronic hypertension or toxemia). In such situations, it is often advantageous to deliver the baby sooner because these babies tend to do better than if they remained in the uterus of a very sick mother. An amniocentesis may also be performed if you go into very early spontaneous labor. Two drugs—ritodrine and terbutaline—are very effective in stopping premature labor. Ritodrine is administered intravenously or subcutaneously. When the mother becomes more stable, the drugs can be taken orally. When the woman is stable on the oral dose, she then may be able to go home on the medication. Oral ritodrine will be continued for as long as it is deemed necessary. Encouragingly, premature labor sometimes is reversible.

If labor cannot be stopped, in order to help prevent RDS, and providing there is sufficient time, a corticosteroid drug may be administered so that when the baby is delivered its lungs will be able to accommodate air passing through them. The effect of corticosteroids lasts from seven to ten days.

Because to date there have been so many repeat and elective cesareans, amniocentesis to determine fetal lung maturity has become increasingly common. Again, spontaneous labor is encouraged above all other measures because, in most instances, this means that the baby is ready to be born. Once the uterus is opened, the doctor cannot say, "Hmm, this baby is having difficulty breathing. I think I'll put her back in for a while." Over the past decade, many expectant mothers have had to undergo amniocentesis.

The longest part of the test is laboratory analysis. At least four hours are required for analysis. Laboratories have different methods of evaluating fetal lung maturity. If the $1/s$ ratio is being determined, they have different scales. In some labs, readings do not exceed 6:1 (6 being the greatest amount of lecithin possible according to their methods). Where other methods and rating scales are used, readings can be as high as 8:1, 10:1, or even 14:1. No matter what method is employed, a reading of 2:1 or higher usually indicates that it is probably safe to schedule the baby's birth within a few days. If a reading of less than 2:1 is taken (for example, 1.5:1), or if the result is close to 2:1 (such as 2.1:1), and there are no other circumstances that would make waiting longer for the baby's birth a problem, the doctor may ask for a second amniocentesis in a week or two, or wait for the onset of labor. The amount of lecithin given off by the baby's lungs can change dramatically within a week's time. The first ratio may have been 1.8:1 and a week later be up to 6:1. Usually, the longer the fetus remains in the mother's uterus, the greater the chances that the infant's lungs will be able to function well on their own.

The results of the 1/s ratio will be eagerly awaited by the parents-to-be if they have a doctor who insists on scheduling repeat and elective cesareans without benefit of labor. When the test results indicate fetal maturity (and as a caution, remember there is some room for error) a cesarean will be scheduled within a few days. Although you have had months to prepare, the very fact that you know when your baby will be born can cause tremendous anxiety. It is not uncommon to feel unprepared, even after all the preparations and waiting. Conversely, the results may indicate that the baby prefers to stay right where she is for at least another week or two. When low 1/s ratios are obtained, then parents may feel very let down. You begin to think your baby will never be born, that you've been pregnant forever, and that the sooner the baby's born, the happier you'll be.

There are three things to remember about amniocentesis to determine fetal lung maturity:

1. It will not tell the sex or chromosomal make-up of the baby. When there is a question regarding genetics, an amniotic tap is done early in the second trimester. Soon this kind of tap will almost certainly be performed in the first trimester.

2. If you go into labor spontaneously shortly after a low 1/s ratio is determined, it is reassuring to note that the spontaneous onset of labor can be beneficial and indicate that the baby's lungs have also readied themselves.

3. Recent research has begun to reveal a previously undiscovered type of respiratory distress associated not so

much with relative fetal maturation as with the mode of delivery itself. Even when ultrasound and 1/s ratios have indicated fetal maturity, there are reports of babies delivered by cesarean ". . . [who] did not have classical respiratory distress, with direct injury to lung tissue, but a condition known as persistent fetal circulation. 'What we *think* happens—no one really knows—is that the blood flow from the right ventricle of the heart to the pulmonary [lung] arteries is inadequate."[2] In other words, there is a greater risk of RDS for babies delivered by cesarean than if they were delivered vaginally. This is another reason for favoring cesarean prevention.

ESTRIOL COUNTS

Estriol is a hormone given off by the fetus, which passes through the placenta and into the mother's urine. An estriol count is a lab test to determine the level of estriol present in your urine. The level of estriol indicates how well the placenta is functioning. When there is a question of postmaturity and the doctor advises that the estriol level be determined, the mother must collect all her urine for a twenty-four-hour period (and the container had better be a big one!). At least two estriol evaluations, spaced over a week to ten days apart, are necessary in order to verify the quantity of estriol present. Estriol evaluations may also be done daily, if necessary. Estriol counts tend to be inaccurate and time-consuming. Because there are now quicker, more reliable tests (such as contraction testing, discussed below), this test is being replaced, though not completely as yet. Estriol testing does have advantages in some pregnancies—and it is noninvasive.

NONSTRESS TESTING

Nonstress testing takes place when there is a question of fetal movement and well-being. This test may be of particular interest to diabetic mothers. It is a simple procedure (too simple and nonconclusive, contend some critics) that requires a mother to have an external fetal monitor placed around her abdomen for a certain period of time (twenty minutes or more). When the baby moves, she presses a button so that the fetal heart rate can be compared to fetal activity. Another alternative to nonstress testing is fetal movement charting (see below).

Some authorities, including Gail Brewer, author of *What Every Pregnant Woman Should Know,*[3] suggest that if there is concern over adequate function of the placenta, instead of undergoing tests the mother should improve her diet during the last weeks of pregnancy to increase blood flow through the placenta. When you have a nonstress test, remember that what you consume prior to the test (including cigarettes and tranquilizers) will influence how much your baby does or does not move. And what happens if your baby chooses that time to take a nap? There won't be any fetal activity for you to note. If this is the case, it is recommended that you eat something sweet to awaken the napping baby.

CONTRACTION OR "STRESS" TESTING

When there is doubt about adequate placental functioning (as may be the case with a woman who has diabetes, renal disease, toxemia, hypertension, or when there is postmaturity or a prolonged absence of fetal movement), a stress test can be given. Although the procedure is the same, this test goes by several different names, including contraction stress testing and oxytocin challenge testing.

For stress testing, you'll be admitted to the hospital and attached to a fetal monitor. An IV (intravenous) will be administered with a sufficient amount of Pitocin (synthetic oxytocin) to produce three strong contractions within a ten-minute period. (The amount of contraction-inducing synthetic hormone will not induce labor, just three strong contractions for a short interval.) If the baby's heartbeat remains good during the contractions, and there are no worrisome decelerations, it means that the baby is doing well and that pregnancy can continue for at least another week without endangering the unborn baby. Should severe fetal distress present itself, a cesarean will be scheduled.

Stress testing is denounced by many naturalists. False readings may be obtained. The stress of the test itself on the mother may in turn affect the fetus. Further, the synthetic hormone used in the test can be avoided altogether. Strong contractions can be brought on with stimulation of the nipples. (You can prove this to yourself if you don't already know it: erotic stimulation during foreplay or after orgasm is almost sure to produce a good round of Braxton Hicks contractions).

If a good fetal heart pattern is determined during the stress test, the mother-to-be can go home. Sometimes stress testing is repeated at weekly intervals for as long as necessary. The objective in cases of mothers and babies who have special problems is to ensure delivery at a time that is optimal for *both* mother and baby. Relaxation breathing exercises will help relieve any tension you're having before and during the test. The contractions will not be severe enough to cause pain or discomfort. The sensation you'll experience will be similar to the Braxton Hicks contractions that are normally felt during the last trimester.

FETAL ACTIVITY CHARTING

Fetal activity or movement charts are simple, non-invasive, and can be done at home. Three times a day at *regularly scheduled times,* stop all your activities. For the next thirty minutes, while you are relaxing, chart the number of movements you feel the baby make. This means kicking, turning around, whatever. The only rigid rule you must follow is that you have to do this at the *same time each day.* This way, you'll be very reassured. Bear in mind that smoking substantially reduces a baby's movements (and contributes to a higher incidence of other problems in pregnancy, including placenta previa), as will smoking marijuana or taking drugs (be they prescription or recreational drugs). This is one of the few pregnancy tests that is noninterventionist and without risk.

BIOPHYSICAL PROFILE

A "biophysical profile" or "biophysical monitoring" is a new antenatal test to determine fetal maturity. Although this test requires use of ultrasound, it avoids the use of contraction testing. Biophysical profiles also eliminate the need for hospitalization to administer contraction-stimulating drugs intravenously and subject mother and baby to a battery of interventions. Usually, a *nonstress* test is required in advance of biophysical monitoring.

In brief, a biophysical profile accomplishes the following: By observing the fetus with ultrasound, a number of observations can be noted—fetal breathing movements, amount of amniotic fluid, placental maturity, fetal muscle tone, and fetal activity. A healthy fetus is active, has a particular regular breathing pattern, and accelerates its heart rate with activity. With good placental function, there is no decrease in amniotic fluid and the placenta is not unusually thin or calcified. A good score on the biophysical profile has been associated with a subsequent healthy baby.

HORMONE TESTING

Estriol is not the only hormone to be measured in some pregnancies, particularly when possible postmaturity is combined with very high blood pressure, when Rh sensitization is suspected, etc. Human placental lactogen (HPL) is made only by the placenta, and its presence in normal concentrations (which increase with every test) indicates that the placenta is doing its work as it should. Evaluation of this hormone can be done by means of a blood test.

TO TEST OR NOT TO TEST,
THAT IS THE QUESTION

Expectant parents are confronted with a series of decisions, which start even before pregnancy commences. Once a woman is pregnant, parents-to-be must decide, among other things, whether she should submit to antenatal tests to determine fetal maturity and well-being. These tests, singly or in combination, are not infallible, but when needed they are better than anything yet devised to help ensure that a baby is born healthy and fully matured. In all likelihood, antenatal tests, employed judiciously and when there are clear signs or circumstances that point to the need to utilize them, may be far more beneficial than risky. Yet the decision to go forward or to refuse such testing is a personal one. As much faith as we place in nature, the fact remains that neither nature nor state-of-the-art medicine is perfect. If we could rely on nature 100 percent of the time, there would never be a miscarriage, stillbirth, or imperfect baby. The newly developed ways to communicate with the unborn baby are far from perfect and only one, fetal activity charting, is without some risk. You must (as always) weigh potential benefit against potential risk. And then you must apply your common sense, personal values and beliefs, and the recommendations of the health care professionals you have chosen in order to decide if you will or will not undergo any one or a combination of these tests.

SIGNS OF LABOR
AND WHAT TO DO

Considering the fact that fewer and fewer cesareans are being scheduled, it is important for parents to know the signs of labor and what to do when it occurs. This means that you should be prepared for the onset of spontaneous labor even if your doctor has stubbornly refused to consider a trial of labor and even if you have one of the very rare problems that contraindicate vaginal delivery. In other words, do not be lulled into thinking you are "immune" to labor. It *can* happen. It may occur weeks before the baby is due, or a few hours before a scheduled cesarean.

The experience of a woman in the Midwest will illustrate the point. She had seen her doctor in the afternoon. He told her that she was doing nicely and that she should check in.o the hospital the next morning for tests. On the way home from the doctor's office, she began to have what she described as a bad backache. By the time she and her husband arrived home, the ache was localized in her lower abdomen and felt like menstrual cramps. She curled up on the couch and put her head on her husband's lap. But she did not call the obstetrician because she didn't want to bother "such a busy man" and because she did not want to call him for something so "trivial" as a few cramps. She thought that if she waited a bit longer, the cramps would go away. When her membranes ruptured and stained their nice white sofa, her husband told her that perhaps she could wait, but he couldn't. He called the doctor. Just over an hour later, she had her baby delivered by cesarean.

All parents should know the signs of labor. They are:

> loss of the mucus plug
> bloody show
> rupture of membranes (breaking of the amniotic sac or "bag of waters")
> contractions
> a combination of any or all of the above

If you go into labor spontaneously and are not expecting it, don't panic. Welcome it. The controversy over rupture of cesarean scars is unfounded. If your doctor does not believe in labor trials and subsequent vaginal deliveries, you may be issued warnings about how spontaneous labor can rupture your old scar. Don't believe these warnings. Even the American College of Obstetrics and Gynecology (of which your obstetrician is probably a member) now freely admits that "although uterine rupture can occur, it is rarely catastrophic with the availability of modern fetal monitoring, anesthesia, and obstetric support services." (For a thorough discussion of subsequent vaginal delivery, uterine scar rupture, etc., see Chapter 16.) In other words, should spontaneous labor begin, you may want to call your doctor immediately, but chances are that a few contractions will not cause any major problems. If, however, your labor starts prematurely, try to determine if the contractions are the "real thing" or just strong Braxton Hicks contractions.

To find out which is which, simply stop what you're doing. If you've been in bed, get up and walk around. If you've been on your feet, lie down on your left side with your knees slightly flexed. Braxton Hicks contractions are felt in varying intensity and with varying frequency after about the seventh month of pregnancy. Thus, if the contractions you're having are of the Braxton Hicks variety, they'll stop or diminish considerably once you've altered your activity. If they're the real thing, these measures will not stop them. If you find that you are having real contractions, call your doctor or midwife immediately. Don't panic, however, because with new drugs, particularly ritodrine, premature labor can almost always be stopped.

BENEFITS OF SPONTANEOUS LABOR

What happens if you go into labor a few days or weeks before the baby is due? Is this dangerous? No—not unless labor occurs very, very early. Spontaneous labor does not necessarily mean a premature baby. Spontaneous labor is nature's way of telling you that this is the time for the baby to be born. The same hormones that trigger labor also stimulate the baby's systems and prepare the baby for life outside the uterus. And it cannot be reiterated enough: contractions almost never rupture a previous uterine incision, nor do they spell catastrophe for either mother or baby.

An ever-increasing number of obstetricians encourage spontaneous labor, even if there are contraindications that rule out vaginal delivery. The most conservative doctors are abandoning the practice of scheduling elective and repeat cesareans. As mentioned, ritodrine has proven remarkably effective in stopping premature labors. However, should it happen that labor cannot be stopped or there are other factors that necessitate quick delivery of the baby, it is reassuring to know that advances in skill and technology within the field of special care for "premies" have greatly improved the chances of survival for premature and at-risk newborns.

Although your time, energy, and finances may be limited, you may want to find a doctor who actively encourages you to wait until labor has started of its own accord before proceeding with a cesarean. You may also want to find a doctor and a hospital where your wishes to attempt subsequent vaginal delivery are actively encouraged. A doctor who gives lip service to your desire may turn out to offer only verbal and insincere support. There are numerous groups throughout the United States and Canada that can help steer you to a doctor and hospital that truly advocate and encourage subsequent vaginal delivery (see "Resources").

Dr. Robert S. Mendelsohn, author of *Confessions of a Medical Heretic* and *Mal(e) Practice,* has this to say about subsequent vaginal delivery:

> Not until 1980, after the Caesarean section rate had tripled in the United States, did the National Institutes of Health issue new guidelines telling doctors that vaginal delivery for women who had previously been sectioned is as safe as, or safer than, another section. The guidelines also urged that when labor contractions are not strong enough women be permitted to move around and exercise to stimulate natural labor. Only after exhausting all other measures should surgery be employed. . . . I will watch with interest to see what effect the new guidelines have. They didn't tell the obstetricians anything they didn't already know, but they certainly tell mothers some things the obstetricians didn't want them to hear. Perhaps they will persuade the doctors to give their scalpels a rest.

Put in its most elemental terms, when labor starts, the only thing you should do is relax. Nature will take care of the rest.

PREPARING FOR THE BIRTH:
HOSPITAL ADMISSIONS
AND ROUTINES

Although many birth activists correctly denounce scheduled cesareans, and I count myself among them, reality must be confronted. In some areas, despite parents' best efforts, it will be impossible (in the foreseeable future, at least) to find a doctor and hospital within reasonable distance, covered by their medical insurer, and otherwise available to them where they can let nature—and not the doctor's schedule or the arbitrary and sometimes incorrect results of antenatal tests— determine the baby's birth day. In addition, there are and always will be exceptional circumstances that dictate the need for a planned cesarean delivery date. Such circumstances are exceedingly infrequent, but they can occur. For example, on May 21, 1985, septuplets (seven babies) were born to Patricia and Samuel Frustaci, of Riverside, California. In order to improve the babies' chances for survival, the hospital had to borrow extra personnel and equipment from other hospitals. A large team of doctors, nurses, and therapists had to be on call to handle the births, which took place by cesarean after twenty- eight weeks of gestation. Each baby was cared for by a neonatologist (a doctor who specializes in the care of preterm and critically ill newborns). In other words, in order to ensure that the babies were brought into the world with a maximal chance of survival, a network of personnel and equipment had to be prepared well in advance. In this and other situations, chances cannot be taken. However, in most cases, this kind of advance preparation is unnecessary, and you should be able to check into the hospital after labor has started or only a few hours before delivery.

Not too long ago, doctors did not even entertain the possibility of vaginal birth after cesarean, nor did they consider waiting to do the cesarean until after labor started. Instead, you were inevitably admitted to the hospital the day before the one decreed by the obstetrician as your baby's date of birth. For most of us, and for those who still must capitulate to this outdated practice, those hours of waiting were endless and anxious. They were also a waste of time and money. Cesarean mothers-to-be are not sick. They are simply going to have a baby, albeit by appointment. It is now increasingly common for the expectant mother to be admitted a few hours before the delivery, rather than a whole day in advance. This policy is better, but it should not be considered preferable to waiting for labor to start. However, if this is the way you must give birth, at least going to the hospital a few hours before the delivery makes it seem more like a birth experience and less like a surgical procedure.

ADMITTING ROUTINES

You will know in advance what time you are expected to check into the hospital. Much of the paperwork can be done beforehand (in the latter weeks of pregnancy) so that the time spent on the actual day of admission will be less. In some hospitals, you will have to register at the reception desk, and then wait until you are called into the admitting office to complete forms that require your name, address, social security number, religion, doctor's name, and the person or company responsible for payment of the bill. It will be necessary to sign a release form (informed consent) stating that you understand what type of procedure(s) you will undergo. If you do not understand exactly what is to be done, find out before you sign the form. Some mothers wish to have a tubal ligation done at the same time as their cesarean if they know they do not want to have more children. Thus the tubal ligation procedure as well as the cesarean will appear on the release form.

When you are officially admitted to the hospital, you will be given an identification bracelet to wear until discharge. It bears your name, address, religion, doctor's name, drug allergies (if any), and a special code number, which you and your baby will share. Once you are admitted, and whether or not you are in labor, many hospitals still insist that you be taken to your room in a wheelchair, even though it is unnecessary.

Your vital signs (pulse, blood pressure, and temperature) will be taken soon after admission, and every few hours thereafter until the birth. Blood samples are drawn so that the lab can do an analysis of your blood type in case transfusion is necessary. About 10 percent of all women giving birth by cesarean will require blood transfusion.

In addition to checks on your vital signs, a respiratory and lung capacity test may be given. This pulmonary function test requires that you breathe into a tube, similar to a vacuum cleaner hose.

In some hospitals, another outdated routine may still be imposed on you: total "prepping" of body hair so that it does not interfere with the incision. Until fairly recently total preps were done as a matter of standard procedure. In such instances, every hair from beneath the breasts, between the legs, and up to the tailbone was shaved. A total prep for cesarean mothers is thoroughly unnecessary, undignified, demeaning, and pointless. A partial prep, which is more common now, is all that is needed, and it is much more comfortable when the hair grows in. For a partial prep, hair is shaved away only from the area where the incision is to be made; this includes a small abdominal area and the hair visible when both legs are together.

Soon after your admission, an anesthesiologist will visit you to inquire about your medical history and your preference for anesthesia. (Types of anesthesia are discussed later in this chapter.) Although much of your medical history is on file with your obstetrician, this visit from the anesthesiologist is a good way of double-checking. The medical history will include questions about allergies, physical debilities, weight, and previous surgical experience. You may be asked what type of anesthesia you prefer (spinal, epidural, or general). It is usually possible to ask for a spinal or epidural; only if there are medical contraindications will you have to have a general. Feel free to ask about the various types available to you. If you have any questions, the anesthesiologist is the person who can answer them. You are not expected to know all the hows and whys of anesthesia.

If you have been admitted to the hospital the day before the baby's birth, a dietician will bring you a menu for supper. No matter how nervous you are, order something nourishing and eat it. It's going to be a long time between this meal and your next one. If dinner comes and it is totally unpalatable, be sure to order something from a restaurant or call home for someone to bring you food. Don't be surprised if you feel a little nervous and queasy. The anticipation of the next day's events are exciting and jitters are to be expected. But try to calm yourself and eat something. If you're at home the night before you're scheduled to have your baby, perhaps you could go out to dinner or enjoy the company of friends to help celebrate (modestly) the next day's event.

If you've been admitted the night before, your obstetrician may drop in for a visit during the evening rounds. Moments before the doctor arrives, you may be on the verge of tears and have hundreds of questions to ask. But the moment your doctor walks in and asks how you are doing, you reply, "Just fine. I had some questions but I can't remember them now." Out goes the doctor and as soon as the door closes you remember what you wanted to say. Always keep a piece of paper and a pen handy to write down your questions and concerns.

Including dinner, the total amount of time that preoperative routines and visits require can be condensed into about an hour. No wonder the recent trend is to wait for spontaneous labor or at least to admit you to the hospital only a few hours before the birth. If you're in the hospital the day before, you may become bored, restless, or very anxious. Most of the hours are spent waiting . . . waiting . . . waiting. You may be the only woman on the maternity floor who is still pregnant. All the other mothers are involved with their babies, receiving visitors, chatting together about their newborns. And there you are, feeling very left out. You may be apprehensive, afraid, worried about the health of your baby, the possible danger of anesthesia and surgery, the responsibilities of caring for a newborn, how older siblings are doing at home without you. If you go for a walk around the floor, you may feel overly self-conscious about your still-pregnant belly. You may even feel jealous and depressed. Much of the trepidation you're feeling may be magnified and translated into acute anxiety because, not only are you a little scared, you may also feel trapped. Knowledge of what to expect and how to prepare for this time of waiting, coupled with the support of your mate and the hospital staff, can alleviate much of your apprehension.

Even when you are admitted to the hospital the night before, some hospitals now offer champagne and candlelight dinners for mothers- and fathers-to-be. At other places, you can check out for a few hours to have dinner at a nearby restaurant, maybe see a movie, and be back in your bed around ten or eleven. If these options are not open to you, prepare in advance for the hours of waiting and worrying. Bring a good book to read, write letters, address birth announcements, or finish a project, such as embroidering a robe for the new baby. Watch television. Make the hospital room more "homey" and personal by decorating it with pictures of your loved ones, a favorite poster, flowers, or some treasure from home that makes you feel more secure. Splurge on a long-distance phone call to someone you haven't seen for ages. Play cards or Trivial Pursuit. Keeping yourself busy will relieve your tension and make the time pass more quickly.

Your husband or a special friend should spend much of this time waiting with you. Don't be surprised if you feel inhibited by the hospital atmosphere. The most important thing is being together. Even if your hospital has twenty-four-hour visiting privileges for fathers, your husband may not want to stay all night unless there's a bed for him there, too. Having a bed for the father is a practice found in many countries around the world, but not yet in the United States. Both you and your mate will benefit from a good night's sleep. It is important that the baby's father or your birth support person has something good to eat before coming back to the hospital the next morning. Being well hydrated and nourished reduces the likelihood of nausea, dizziness, and fainting.

For women admitted the day prior to birth, after midnight you'll be NPO (a Latin abbreviation for "nothing by mouth"). If you have never craved a snack in the wee hours of the night, this is one time in your life when you may become extra thirsty or hungry, probably because you're tense and excited and possibly simply because you know you can't have anything to eat or drink. If you want, however, have a light snack around 10 or 11 P.M. Forbidding food and drink eight hours before delivery is the precaution taken to reduce the risk of obstructing the breathing passages with vomitus while under anesthesia. However, it is still entirely possible that with spinal or epidural anesthesia you may feel sick to your stomach even though you've had nothing to eat or drink for many hours prior to the delivery.

During the evening while you wait out the hours until it is time for the baby to be born, you may have difficulty sleeping. That's perfectly natural. If you're offered a sleeping pill, it is *not* recommended that you take it since it will cross the placenta and may linger in the baby's tissue for weeks after birth. If you cannot sleep, call upon your resources to relax, or, failing that, read, watch TV, talk with your spouse or support person, etc. The floor nurses should be willing to spend some time with you. Even if they do nothing but listen, having someone with whom to share a few minutes of your thoughts and worries will reduce your anxiety.

Slowly (too slowly), the medical tradition of scheduling cesareans and requiring that mothers be admitted the day prior to the birth is being abandoned. Meanwhile, this is still the case in certain areas and, as mentioned, there will always be special circumstances in which such practice may be required.

ANESTHESIA

An *anesthesiologist* is a doctor who has had special training in the field of anesthesia. This doctor decides the type and amount of anesthesia to be given and is able to administer it independently. An *anesthetist* is a highly trained nurse who learns to identify and recognize patient problems that can affect the plan and course of anesthetic management. The type, amount, and monitoring of anesthesia is done under the supervision of a physician. These two terms are often confusing to the lay person.

Three types of anesthesia are used for cesarean childbirth: spinal, epidural, and general. With spinals and epidurals, mothers are awake and aware for their babies' births. Pain is eliminated, although some minor sensation may be experienced. With general anesthesia, the mother is put to sleep and is unaware of what is happening until an hour or more after delivery. (The types of anesthesia are described in more detail below.) The type of anesthesia used for delivery depends on several factors:

1. Your medical history.

2. The preference of your doctor and/or the anesthesia department. Sometimes the type of anesthesia used depends on who is available in the anesthesia department when the cesarean takes place. Smaller community hospitals, unlike major medical centers, do not always keep round-the-clock teams of anesthesiologists on duty. The person called in may influence the type of anesthesia you have. For this reason, make it your business to find out in advance if all anesthesia options are open to you at all times. This is especially important if you have your heart set on being awake for your baby's birth and there are no medical contraindications for spinal or epidural anesthesia.

3. Trends in obstetric anesthesia. They are subject to change, so even if you had general anesthesia with a prior birth, you may still be able to have a spinal or epidural this time. It's important to ask questions about anesthesia in advance of delivery, especially if you are having this baby at a different hospital or with a different doctor.

There has been some debate among medical professionals about general anesthesia (something most cesarean parents do *not* want, barring medical contraindications). Doctors who favor general anesthesia have cited the fact that it may reduce the possibility of *hypotension*. Hypotension is a condition that may develop as a result of a reduction in the patient's blood pressure, which, if it takes place, will occur very shortly after anesthesia has been administered. With spinal or epidural anesthesia, some mothers (especially if they are tense or fearful, and sometimes even if they are not) may become dizzy or nauseated. Intravenous prehydration will relieve temporary feelings of dizziness or nausea and is a small price to pay for being able to see, hear, and touch one's baby within seconds of birth. If there is some medical contraindication that precludes the possibility of spinal or epidural anesthesia for your delivery, your doctor should discuss these openly and honestly with you.

I feel (and other parents and professionals join me in this view) that mothers should be allowed a choice of anesthesia. This is especially important if you give birth in a hospital where cesareans are still almost always being performed with general anesthesia. Most parents prefer spinals or epidurals.

4. Regional bias. This means that certain geographic parts (regions) of the country seem to follow a pattern in what kind of anesthesia is available to the community.

5. Time element. A very, very few cesareans are emergency emergencies, in which it is a dire necessity to get the baby out as quickly as possible. In such cases, there may be no choice but to use the type of anesthesia most quickly available.

6. The final and most important consideration is the mother herself. For a first-time emergency cesarean, the mother may be exhausted after a trying labor and request general anesthesia. She may be afraid that there will be additional stress and pain if she chooses to have a spinal or epidural. Because mothers-to-be are not always well versed in how a cesarean takes place, they may think that they will hear, see, or feel something awful. There are also a few women who are told, or suspect, that their babies' lives are endangered, or who dread the thought of seeing a baby born who is deformed. They may opt for general anesthesia as a sort of self-protection to avoid knowing what happens to them and their babies until they are better able to cope.

By and large, most mothers want to see their babies at birth. Any initial misgivings or fears can be overcome with support and information from the mother's obstetrician, her anesthesiologist, her nurses, and her husband. With education and empathy come confidence: the cesarean mother will know what to expect and how to cope effectively without panic. Being awake for the baby's birth enables the mother to initiate the maternal-infant bonding processes and to rejoice in the baby's arrival.

General Anesthesia. General anesthesia can be given either by placing a mask over the mother's nose and mouth or inserting a needle into her arm. With either method, the mother-to-be becomes unconscious within a few seconds. She will remember nothing until an hour or more after delivery, when she groggily awakens. Women sometimes report that they awaken thinking they are still in labor. Some of these mothers find it hard to believe that their babies have been born, especially if they have also been separated from them for many hours.

The myth that all cesareans must be performed with general anesthesia is persistent and perpetuated partially by some obstetricians and partially by the lack of information with which cesarean parents have had to contend. It is difficult to make an intelligent decision based on myth and misinformation. When a mother chooses to have general anesthesia, one of her reasons (in fact, the primary one) may be fear: fear of the unknown, fear of possible pain, or the trauma of a previous cesarean birth, which makes the thought of being awake anathema to her.

Another reason why some women have general anesthesia is that they are unaware of the alternatives. If the mother has had an opportunity to discuss her anxieties with someone who is able to relate to her experiences, it is not surprising to have her change her mind and ask for a spinal or epidural, rather than general anesthesia. The anesthesiologist is of course a prime source of information and support, but unfortunately, most expectant mothers do not meet with an anesthesiologist until the night before they are to deliver. Therefore, the responsibility of informing parents of the options lies with the obstetrician who sees the mother throughout pregnancy. The mother should feel free to ask questions of her doctor as they come up, and, it is hoped, have her fears set to rest. Also, the support and empathy that another woman or another cesarean mother is able to give are often an added bonus.

Spinals and Epidurals. Spinals and epidurals share the benefit of allowing mothers to be awake, aware, and comfortable for the birth. They reduce the potential negative effects of general anesthesia, which may sometimes cross the placenta and depress the baby's systems. Although spinals are more commonly used than epidurals, the type given depends on many things, including your doctor's preference, the hospital's location, and preexisting medical conditions, such as high or low blood pressure or severe back problems that would make it difficult, if not impossible, to successfully administer these anesthetics.

Both spinals and epidurals are administered to the patient's back. The epidural takes effect more slowly than the spinal, and additional medication is given during the delivery by means of a catheter (a thin tube), which is kept in place during the delivery. The spinal is given by means of injecting a small quantity of medication in the back just once. It is done just a few minutes before the obstetrician is ready to deliver the baby. Both create a temporary paralysis (numbing) from the chest to the tips of the toes. There is usually no sensation whatsoever, but the mother may feel pressure as the baby is actually being delivered. Pressure, pulling, or tugging sensations, which herald the baby's imminent arrival, are discussed in more detail in Chapter 8.

Other Forms of Anesthesia. Although there are other forms of anesthesia, they are not widely accepted or used in the United States. Acupuncture is frequently used in China; Shirley MacLaine's film *China: The Other Half of the Sky* shows a cesarean birth taking place with acupuncture as the sole means of anesthesia. The mother is smiling, eating bits of fruit fed to her by a nurse, and waves at the camera. Acupuncture has been used for several cesarean births in the United States.

Some experimentation with hypnosis has been done in this country. A film produced some years ago for physicians shows a Midwestern cesarean mother who is having her third cesarean delivery under hypnosis. It is obvious that the woman and her obstetrician have worked closely in preparation for the delivery. During the delivery, the mother sings as a means of taking her mind away from what is happening. The doctor suggests that the room is very warm—despite the fact that it is quite cool. The woman is told to open her eyes and look at her baby before she is again placed in a "trance" so that suturing can be done. In an interview soon after the delivery, she remembers no pain, but she does recall that the delivery room was very warm and that she wanted a cool drink to make herself more comfortable.

As anesthetic alternatives, acupuncture and hypnosis are interesting to note, and do emphasize the fact that mind over matter often is an essential key to the reduction of discomfort.

Making the Choice. I want to encourage women to have anesthesia that will permit them to be awake for the birth of their babies. However, before making the decision (when there *is* a choice) it is advisable to weigh the pros and cons and to consider the possible benefits and risks of each type of anesthesia. A woman who is deeply fearful may be better off having general anesthesia. If you're afraid to have a spinal or epidural because you're terrified of what you'll hear or see, you might do well to talk to cesarean parents who have experienced childbirth with either of these types of anesthesia. Very often, their experiences—even if they were not smooth and perfect— will do much to convince you to change your mind.

The real benefits of spinal or epidural anesthesia are often enumerated in human, rather than medical, terms. The cesarean delivery *is* the birth of a baby. You'll want to participate in the birth, to feel a part of what is going on. Even if you can't deliver vaginally, at least with spinal or epidural anesthesia you'll be able to hear your baby's first cries and will see your infant within seconds after birth. You will also be able to establish eye contact with your baby, hold him or her, and reassure yourself that the baby is well. This promotes mother-infant bonding and attachment processes and may help you feel more like a mother sooner. It's also a wonderful time of rejoicing shared with your husband or support person, who'll be there to comfort you and witness this wonderful event. This does not mean that you're a bad mother if you have general anesthesia, or that you may turn out to be less motherly. What it does mean is simple: being comfortable and awake for the birth and seeing your newborn within seconds will almost certainly make it easier for you to finalize your pregnancy and initiate your role as parent. If you have general anesthesia because of medical conditions (such as back injury or blood pressure problems), or because it is the only type of anesthesia available where you deliver, rest assured that as long as you are highly motivated (which you probably are), you will relate well to your baby and overcome the odds. Because hospitals now almost always permit the father and/or a support person to be present for the birth, even when the mother has general anesthesia, that person will be able to cuddle and hold the baby within minutes of birth even if you cannot. Knowing that someone close to you is right beside you (perhaps taking pictures to show you later), and that your baby will be welcomed into the world by a loving daddy or friend can help make up for what you and the baby missed.

HOW TO MAKE THE ADMINISTRATION OF ANESTHESIA EASIER

In rare cases of an emergency cesarean, there is not enough time to choose the type of anesthesia used. During subsequent pregnancies, however, cesarean mothers may be very apprehensive about anesthesia. One of their anxieties is the actual administration of the anesthetic. To make the administration of a spinal or epidural easier, for both you and the anesthesiologist, here are some suggestions on how to cope effectively.

Administration of anesthesia requires just a few minutes. During this period you will want to be as relaxed, comfortable, and confident as possible.

If the baby's father or a support person is to be present for the birth, he or she may be asked to wait outside the delivery room until after you have been given the anesthesia, or if permitted to stay in the room, may have to sit off to the side for this procedure. While preparations are being made, a way to break tension is to converse with the anesthesiologist, your obstetrician, the delivery room nurses, your husband, or your support person. The obstetrician will be in the room by this time, because your doctor will want to begin the delivery very soon after the anesthesia has taken effect. It is helpful to establish eye contact with someone in the room, and that someone should be the baby's father or your support person. You're going to have a baby, and looking at someone whose presence is familiar and comforting is more reassuring than staring at the ceiling or the drapes.

For administration of the anesthesia, you'll be asked to sit up or turn on your side and bring your knees up to your chin. You need to bend as much as possible. After your knees are flexed or you are bent forward, you may experience a momentary panic attack. Discipline and relaxation breathing techniques will help. Think of your body as a rainbow and arch your back toward the anesthesiologist. Arching serves to separate and make more visible the bones of the spine, and this makes it easier for the doctor to inject the anesthetic. Some anesthesiologists encourage mothers to "arch your back like a mad cat." A mad cat is a tense cat, and because relaxation is important for this step, the image of a rainbow is really preferable because it is more soothing. (There are many reasons why pregnant women are advised to keep their weight within reasonable limits. One of them is that the anesthesiologist may have a harder time finding the "landmarks" of the spine and the introduction of anesthesia may take longer than is necessary. Also, if there is a thick layer of fat between the abdomen and the uterus, it will take longer for the obstetrician to reach the uterus and then to suture all those extra layers.)

You will probably feel something cool being applied to your back before the anesthetic is injected. This bright reddish orange liquid is an antiseptic solution. You will not be able to see your back being cleansed, obviously, but it helps if your spouse or support person knows that the antiseptic may be very colorful. After the antiseptic solution has been applied, you may feel a stinging sensation as a Novocain-like drug is injected. The important thing to remember is that this part of the procedure, which often causes great anxiety, is also very brief. Knowing what is happening and that it will be over soon will help you cope.

Although you may have had to wait for the delivery room to be free, the doctors to arrive, and the room to be set up, once the anesthesia has been given, it will be just five or ten minutes until your baby is born. From here on in, the teamwork and precision of the staff, and the knowledge that you will soon see, hear, and touch your baby, should be comforting—and, it is hoped, this will be a fulfilling, enjoyable experience.

TYPES OF SKIN INCISIONS

Generally when parents talk about incisions, they are referring to the skin incision only. Actually, the obstetrician needs to make a series of incisions, not just one, to reach the uterus. The skin incision is the only visible one, and is often referred to by cesarean mothers as "the scar." There are two types of skin incisions. The vertical midline abdominal incision extends from just below the navel to the top of the pubic bone. The *transverse incision,* often referred to as a "bikini cut," goes from side to side just above the pubic bone. Its cosmetic advantage is that once the pubic hair regrows, it is barely visible.

Which type of skin incision you have will depend on:

1. The time element involved. Sometimes doctors use a classic incision for an emergency cesarean because it may save time, although midline incisions are being abandoned almost entirely.

2. Your doctor's preference. Some doctors feel more comfortable using one type of incision rather than the other. However, it is hoped that when a cesarean must be performed, you have a doctor who prefers and uses a transverse "bikini" incision.

3. Sometimes the mother's preference. Electing the bikini incision is not always possible, especially in those rare instances when time is of the essence.

In recent years, the transverse incision has gained in popularity among medical professionals and mothers. If yours is a repeat cesarean, the new incision can be made at the same location as the old one or, if you had a midline incision previously, this time you may want to ask for a bikini cut. Women who have had both types of incisions report that it is much easier and less painful to recover from a transverse incision.

It is also important to note that no matter which type of skin incision you have, the uterine incision is almost always transverse (horizontal, from side to side, in the lower uterine segment). Today it is thought that the classic uterine incision (vertical, up and down) may weaken the uterus. As a general rule, almost all of today's cesareans take place with a lower-segment uterine incision.

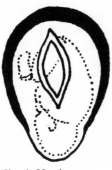 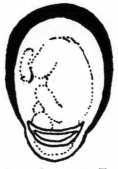

Classic Uterine
Incision

Lower Segment or Transverse
Uterine Incision

BIRTHDAY!

At last! This is the day! All the waiting, wondering, and worrying will soon be past. Finally the baby you have been carrying for nine months will be revealed. You will be able to see, hold, love, cuddle, and kiss your baby. You will soon know if it is a boy or a girl. You will be able to see if the baby has inherited your hair, your husband's eyes, or Grandma's nose. But before all these things can happen, you and your baby will undergo a series of complex steps. The quality of the birth experience, the way you, the parents, will relate to the baby, and how soon you recover will depend on what happens during the baby's birth. If you feel relaxed, confident, and informed, this will be a beautiful day for you, and a time in which the roots of love are planted.

There should be time for you to take a shower before donning a hospital gown called a "johnny." This is one of those garments that is always too big, ties in the back, and is anything but fashionable—but it is efficient. Your husband and/or support person should be allowed to come to the hospital several hours before the scheduled delivery. He or she may walk into your room carrying the morning paper, and hiding behind a self-conscious smile that betrays an air of assurance.

He or she, too, is feeling a little nervous and eager. This morning is a little like a surprise party that you found out about in advance. You won't be surprised by the party, but you will be delighted with the present.

Although each person's experience is unique, the following is a general outline of what you can expect.

Enemas used to be routine preoperative procedures. Although they are now an outdated routine, it wouldn't be at all surprising if a few hospitals still insist upon giving them.

A Foley catheter will be inserted into the urethra (the duct by which urine is discharged from the bladder). Catheterization may take place in your room, if you've been preadmitted, or in the operating room. Insertion is not painful, but some women report that it can be uncomfortable. If you find yourself tense or uncomfortable, relaxation breathing should help. Insertion usually takes just a few seconds. Once the catheter is properly in place, you probably won't feel it at all. How long the catheter remains in place depends on doctor's orders and the mother's condition. Until recently, the catheter was often left in place for twenty-four hours. Today, the catheter is usually removed shortly after delivery. The Foley catheter has two purposes. The immediate one is to drain the bladder and keep it compressed and out of the doctor's way while the baby is being delivered. The other is to eliminate the mother's need to urinate into a bedpan or get out of bed to go to the bathroom. Infections can occur, and the chances of infection increase the longer the catheter is in place.

Formerly doctors ordered that a tranquilizer be injected into the mother shortly before she was taken to the delivery room. This is not routine now but even if offered, it is advisable not to accept this medication. Tranquilizers may, in fact, have a deleterious effect on the baby. Drugs such as Nembutal and Valium are seldom if ever given to a laboring woman an hour or so before delivery since drugs pass quickly through the placenta and into the baby. Cesarean babies who have not had the beneficial stimulation of labor may be unnecessarily "zapped" and "slowed down" if tranquilizers are used shortly before birth. Neither the mother's body nor the baby's will have time to metabolize and assimilate this medication. Cesarean babies do not need this extra burden. Rather than take a chance of depressing the baby's system, cesarean mothers may wish to refuse this medication.

The best preoperative tranquilizers for a cesarean mother are the presence of the baby's father or other support person to reassure her and the confidence that comes from knowing what to expect and how to cope calmly and effectively.

In a few hospitals, the cesarean mother-to-be is allowed to walk from her room to a labor room or directly into the delivery room. Both a nurse and the baby's father accompany her. She is not "ill" in the conventional sense, and if she has not been dosed with a tranquilizer, it helps to make the experience seem more like a birth and less like a standard surgical procedure. If walking is not permitted, a wheelchair rather than a stretcher may be used.

Whether she is taken to the cesarean delivery room (or, in some hospitals, the regular operating suite) by stretcher or wheelchair or is allowed to walk, there will be sufficient time for the mother and her partner to share a few moments together, encouraging each other, hugging and kissing—or crying. The tears that come just before delivery are often a combination of happiness and nervous release. If the father or support person is not permitted to be present for the birth, this is when he or she will be asked to wait in the waiting room or lobby, or to sit in an empty labor room or in the hallway just outside the delivery suite, depending on hospital policy. It is now common for the father or support person to be present for the birth, but even so many hospitals will ask him or her to wait outside for a few minutes while preoperative preparations are made and anesthesia given. Sometimes this waiting period is lengthy. Each doctor, each nurse, and every piece of equipment must be in place before the delivery can begin. Sometimes obstetricians are late. Sometimes the cesarean delivery room is not free when the birth is scheduled. Find out approximately how long the wait will be, so your partner won't panic and think that they have started without him or her. It may take as long as 30 minutes to "set up."

In the delivery room, the mother will be the center of a flurry of activity. Once on the operating table, there is much to be done. Although the order of events may vary, these are some of the things that will happen:

One arm will have a blood pressure cuff wrapped around it, so that your blood pressure can be monitored as often as needed. In the other arm, the anesthesiologist will start an IV (intravenous). The IV will keep the mother hydrated and nourished during the procedure, and perhaps for hours or days thereafter. The IV is also an important emergency route should additional drugs or a blood transfusion be necessary. The amount of blood loss during a cesarean is usually only about a pint. If there is greater bleeding, blood will be administered through this IV. Starting the IV before the delivery begins will make the mother less apt to become hypotensive. Her blood pressure will remain more stable if she has the benefits of extra liquids in advance of delivery, and she will probably not experience some of the side effects associated with anesthesia.

The arm with the blood pressure cuff will be placed at your side. Sometimes the arm remains free; at other hospitals, it is tucked in at your side. More and more, as health care professionals realize how important it is for mothers and babies (and fathers and babies) to touch each other immediately after birth, women's arms are being kept free so that the mother can hold her baby within moments after birth.

As soon as the anesthesia has been given (we will assume it is either a spinal or an epidural), the mother will be quickly turned on her back. This serves to spread the anesthesia equally. Although she may be unaware of it, the operating table will be tilted slightly to the side (usually the left) or a wedge will be placed under her back. This is to take the pressure of the relaxed uterus off the vena cava (the major vein from the lower extremities). Shortly after anesthesia has been given, the abdomen relaxes and spreads out slightly. If the full weight of the uterus and the fetus are not taken off the vena cava, the weight would interfere with the mother's circulation and might produce shortness of breath, a lowering of the blood pressure (which might cause nausea or dizziness), and/or decreased blood supply to the uterus.

After the anesthesia has been given, a number of things will be done so quickly that the mother may be unaware of them. Little disks will be placed on her chest, with wires running to an electrocardiograph (EKG), which records her heartbeat. Displaying the beat on a screen, a line goes up and down with more or less rhythmic bleeps emitted. Quite frequently, the stickers (the little sensory suction cups placed on the mother's chest) become unstuck. When this happens, if you are at all aware of the bleeps, you may wonder what went wrong. Most likely, there is nothing to worry about. Probably the leads from the chest to the machine came off, or the machine malfunctioned. When I had my son, Jon, I was so drugged, exhausted, and overwhelmed by labor that when the bleeping stopped and the line on the screen went flat, I was panic-stricken. I thought I was going into cardiac arrest or was on the verge of death. Since no one in the room (and it seemed as though there were at least a dozen people there) was paying any attention to me, it was only after the anesthesiologist saw the terror on my face that he smiled, replaced the sensory disks, and told me not to worry. I laugh about this incident now, but at the time it was frightening.

An anesthesia screen may also be placed just below the mother's neck. Her gown is draped over it and is covered by another sterile sheet. Its major purpose is to keep the mother from breathing on and thus contaminating the sterile field, but it blocks her view, so that all she will be able to see are the areas on her side, the drape in front of her, and the ceiling above. If you want to see what is happening below the drapes, it is sometimes possible to look into the overhead light. Women who wish to watch their babies being born by cesarean can ask for mirrors like the ones used for vaginal deliveries. Ten or fifteen years ago, using a mirror for vaginal deliveries was considered as outrageous and farfetched as it sometimes is for cesarean mothers today. The refusal of a mirror is often well-intentioned, but having one is an option to which cesarean mothers are entitled. Women who don't want to see what is happening won't ask for a mirror, and a woman who has requested a mirror and becomes uneasy with what she sees can avert her eyes. If a cesarean mother has prior knowledge of what to expect and the desire to watch her baby being born, there is no reason to deny her a mirror.

Also as part of the preparations made for the delivery, a nurse or the obstetrician will apply an antiseptic solution to the mother's abdomen and partway down her legs. It has a rusty, iodine color, and to the uninitiated it may look as though the abdomen has been painted with blood. Sterile drapes, often made of paper, are then placed over the entire lower portion of the mother's body, leaving only the area immediately surrounding the incision site visible.

If nausea, dizziness, or vomiting are to occur, they will probably happen within a few minutes after the anesthesia has been given. Nausea, dizziness, or vomiting *may* happen no matter how long it has been since you last ate, no matter how quickly you are turned, no matter how much the table is tilted, and no matter how calm, cool, and collected you are! It is something that happens *sometimes*. It does not happen to everyone. Panic is the worst reaction to have. If it happens to you, the *first* thing to do is to tell the anesthesiologist, who will give you a little tray to throw up in and/or may give you additional intravenous medication if necessary.

Oxygen is an excellent way to combat these feelings of nausea or dizziness. The oxygen mask may be made of disposable plastic material or of black rubber. The smell of the rubber mask may come from the rubber itself or from traces of the odor of other gases for which it has been used. The mask is sterilized before each use, but the odd smell may linger. Don't panic and think that the anesthesiologist is trying to pull a fast switch and knock you out. When the mask is in place, take big, deep breaths of oxygen for as long as you need it. Extra oxygen will bring almost immediate relief.

When all these preparations have been completed, it is time for the birth of your baby. First-time, emergency cesarean mothers who have been in labor for many hours may have little recollection of just how long the actual delivery took. Repeat cesarean mothers may be acutely aware of each second that passes. It is comforting and useful to know that the amount of time between the introduction of anesthesia and the delivery of the new baby is usually just five to fifteen minutes. How long it takes is a matter of the doctor's speed (some doctors take just a few minutes to reach the baby; others, no less skillful, may take a little longer); how heavy the mother is (it takes extra time to cut through layer after layer of fat); what position the baby is in; what type of anesthesia is used; and what the indication is for the delivery ("emergency" emergencies, such as abruptio placenta, necessitate the greatest speed, while other indications may permit the doctor to work somewhat more slowly). Generally, though, it takes five to fifteen minutes. The doctor will work as quickly as possible no matter what the circumstances. It is necessary to deliver the baby rapidly to reduce the potentially dangerous effects of anesthesia to the fetus. After the baby has been delivered, the pace can be more leisurely, less pressured.

An incision into the skin is first made. The incision is then retracted (pulled back) to reveal the layers beneath the skin. There are layers of subcutaneous fat, the fascia (a tough membrane), abdominal muscles, and the peritoneum (a thin membrane protecting the abdominal cavity and the organs in it). Once these layers have been incised (including dissecting the bladder from the uterus), the doctor can see the uterus, which is a royal purple color. An incision is then made in the wall of the uterus. The transverse (side to side) incision, which is made in the lower part of the uterus, is surprisingly short: three or four inches across is about average. As the uterus is opened, the amniotic fluid may gush out, showering the doctors. If the amniotic sac is intact, the doctor will pierce it and suction the fluid out. At this time there may be a whooshing noise which sounds almost like the little tube the dentist places in your mouth to extract fluids. When you hear this noise, it means that it's almost time for the baby to be born.

When retracted, the three- or four-inch opening in the uterus is about the same size as a fully dilated cervix (ten centimeters). To remove the baby through this relatively small opening, it is sometimes necessary for the obstetrician or the assisting physician to exert pressure on the top of the uterus. This is called fundal pressure. Some women report that they can feel this pressure or pulling. It is not painful, but the surprise element of it may cause a woman to panic, to think that the anesthesia has not taken effect properly. If it happens to you, don't panic. First tell the doctor that you are having this sensation. Second, relaxation and/or dissociative breathing may help. Third, and *most important,* remember that if you do feel this pressure, it is a *good* sign. It means that your baby will be born within a few seconds or minutes at most. This sensation heralds your baby's birth.

How can you tell if it's going to happen to you? You can't. First time, emergency cesarean mothers, especially those who deliver after labor has begun, may be exhausted. "I was so worn out the first time, they could have run over me with a Mack truck and I wouldn't have known the difference" is a typical reaction. The second time around, the cesarean mother has probably been scheduled for delivery. She is not fatigued as a result of labor, and her senses may be especially keen.

Before, during, and after the birth, it is vitally necessary, comforting, and helpful for the doctors and nurses to talk *with* the mother—especially if the father or support person is not beside her. The mother should be asked what *she* wants to talk about. Some mothers prefer a running commentary given by the obstetrician, "I've made the skin incision. . . . Now I've reached the peritoneum. . . . I can see the uterus now. . . . Here comes the baby's head, now the shoulders. . . . Just a few more seconds and we'll see if this little one is a boy or a girl. . . ."

It would be nice to be able to say that the days of doctors and nurses talking about the mother, rather than with and to her, are gone. It would be even nicer to be able to say that doctors are no longer indulging in conversations with each other about fishing trips, French restaurants, or Colonial architecture. Unfortunately, such a statement would be fallacious.

The mother should be made to feel as though she is a woman giving birth, rather than a hunk of flesh being operated on. This is the birth of a baby, not a chat in a country club sauna. The mother and her baby should be the only topics of discussion, unless the mother herself wants to talk about other things. Talking among doctors during surgery is often a way for them to relieve their own tension. If the mother has had general anesthesia, it really doesn't matter what they say to each other, but when the anesthesia is given, a nurse or the baby's father should hold the mother's hand and reassure her until she is asleep. The mother who is awake for the birth of her baby should not be degraded and demoralized. (One mother said, "For all the attention they paid to me they could just as well have unscrewed my head from my torso and taken only my trunk into the delivery room." Another woman commented, "I felt just like the woman in a magic show. My head was at one end of a box, and my feet were sticking out the other end. It seemed as though there were miles in between my head and my body.")

Conversing with the mother will relieve both her own and the doctors' tension and will make her feel like a woman giving birth, rather than an incidental object in the room. When the father or support person is present for the birth, he or she can comfort the mother, describe to her what is happening, and reassure her that all is well.

The size of the delivery room is sometimes a surprise to parents who are familiar only with the huge amphitheaters pictured on television. Large teaching hospitals do have huge delivery rooms, with balconies for observation, but most community hospital delivery rooms (whether they are regular operating rooms or a special cesarean room within the delivery suite) are far smaller. No matter how small, there will always be room for one more, very important person: the father or another special person.

The father or support person is required to wear a scrub suit, mask, and cap and will be asked to either sit or stand beside the mother's head. If seated, his or her view will be almost as limited as the mother's, and it will be the doctor who announces the arrival and sex of the baby. Fathers or other support people who are allowed to stand can see and will be able to make this announcement.

If the baby is lying in the normal position (head down), the top of the baby's head will be the first thing the doctor sees once the uterus has been opened. If the baby is in the breech position, the buttocks are the first visible body part. When the uterus is open, the doctor will reach inside and pull the baby out by hand. Forceps are occasionally used, but these are employed less often nowadays. As soon as the baby's head is out, the doctor or assistant will suction the mucus from the baby's nose and mouth. At this point, you may hear the baby's first cries. And what a beautiful sound! If the baby has a large quantity of mucus, the first cry may sound more like a gurgle. Hearing that cry, your first question may be, "What is it? Is it a boy or a girl?" If the doctor's reply is, "I don't know yet," the parents may be bewildered—unless they know there is a short period between delivery of the baby's head and its body. When the umbilical cord is long enough, the doctor may hold the baby up for the mother to see, while the cord is still attached and the baby is all wet and covered with vernix (a creamy protective substance). This sight will be just as every parent pictures it. It will look just like the films and photos of babies who are delivered vaginally, and who are shown to their mothers a split second after they have emerged. Brand new babies are bluish in color. As the oxygen reaches the body, the baby will gradually "pink up." Because of their distance from the heart, the last part of the baby's body to turn pink will be the hands and feet. The newborn may react to birth in a manner similar to a shadowboxer, as she uncurls from the fetal position. This is both good and healthy. After nine months in the mother's warm, dark, watery world, the bright lights of the delivery room, the relative coolness of its temperature, and the initial "shock" of suddenly having to function and breathe on her own stimulate her body. Soon the baby has been delivered, the umbilical cord will be clamped and cut.

After holding the baby up for the mother (and the father or support person) to see, the baby will be placed in the arms of a nurse, a pediatrician, or the father. Some nurses bring the naked baby immediately over to the mother to see. Then the baby is quickly placed in a specially equipped basinette, which is placed under warming lights similar to the type which keep food hot in restaurants. Additional oxygen will be given to the baby through a tiny mask to ensure an adequate supply of this vitally important substance, and mucus will be suctioned from her nose and mouth. (Cesarean babies, because they have not been squeezed through the birth canal, often have more mucus than babies delivered vaginally.) The baby's Apgar score, a quick, simple rating of the newborn's reflexes (see chart on next page), will be taken at one and five minutes after birth. The rating system was developed by Dr. Virginia Apgar as a standardized way to record infants' reflexes. A score of 8 or higher indicates a healthy baby. Mild problems may be present in babies with an Apgar of between 5 and 7. Below 5 means that the baby will need immediate, intensive care.

Apgar Rating System

Sign: Score:	0	1	2
Color	blue, pale	body pink, limbs blue	completely pink
Respiratory effort	absent	slow, irregular, weak cry	strong cry
Heart rate	absent	slow, less than 100	over 100
Muscle tone	limp	some flexation of limbs	active movement
Reflex response to flicking foot	absent	facial grimace	cry

The mother and father have waited a long time for the baby to be born. This is the moment they have anticipated eagerly and occasionally agonized over. Seeing a new baby is an extraordinarily beautiful, awe-inspiring, spiritual sight. This is why it is important for the doctor or nurse to hold the baby for viewing by the mother within seconds of delivery, and why it is infinitely preferable for the baby care unit to be placed within the mother's sight.

If the baby care unit is out of the mother's field of vision, hearing her baby cry will not reassure her that all is well until she can actually see for herself. Although the immediate ministrations to the baby take just a few minutes, those minutes pass like hours. "Is the baby all right?" "What does she look like?" "Is she *really* okay?" "If she's as healthy as you say she is, why can't I see her?" These are questions maternity nurses have heard frequently. Placing the baby care unit where the mother can see is so simple, so obvious, and so right that it is a wonder it took this long to move the units so mothers can see their babies being cared for immediately after birth.

As soon as the infant is cared for, she should be brought directly to the mother or placed in the father's arms. He can then hold the baby close to the mother's face for cuddling, nuzzling, and kissing. Eye and body contact between mothers and babies is now recognized as an essential in providing a good start for bonding. In some hospitals, cesarean mothers are even able (with a little help) to nurse their babies while the remainder of the procedure takes place.

If the baby must be taken out of the delivery room and into the nursery, she should always be presented to the mother and father first. Parents frequently complain that their babies are whisked away. Even if the baby is truly endangered, a brief glance and a kiss on the cheek are preferable to not seeing the baby at all. When the parents have not been able to see the newborn, they may imagine problems far worse than the reality. Most cesarean babies are healthy and perfect. To help keep their babies beside them, some parents hire pediatricians to be present at the time of delivery to ensure that the infant will be well tended to, yet kept close to the parents. Recent studies indicate that even if a baby is severely ill or later succumbs to illness, the grieving process for the parents is less traumatic if they have seen their baby. Almost without exception, the newly delivered cesarean baby can and should be immediately brought to the parents.

While the baby is being cared for and presented to the parents, the obstetrician will begin the final stages of the cesarean procedure. The placenta must be delivered. Usually this large, veined organ comes out intact, and the obstetrician makes certain that it is delivered fully before suturing (sewing up the incision). Suturing is the longest part of the cesarean delivery and may require anywhere from fifteen to forty minutes. If the mother is absorbed in her baby, she will probably be totally unaware of what is happening—at least until the baby leaves the room, if she must. There is no need to hurry with the suturing. The doctor will suture the uterus, the layers of tissue and fiber in the abdominal cavity, and the skin of the abdomen. If the mother has elected to have her tubes tied, the doctor will do so before closing the abdominal cavity. Women who do not wish to have more children find this an excellent occasion for tubal ligation. The abdomen is already opened, so time, money, and effort are saved and the stress of an additional operation avoided.

The internal stitches will be dissolvable. The skin sutures (about 18-20) may be either dissolvable or nonabsorbable. Clamps or staples, rather than stitches, are sometimes used. Nonabsorbable stitches need to be removed on or about the fourth or fifth day. If you are still hospitalized, the stitches will be removed before your discharge. Many women are discharged on the third to fifth postpartum day, and in such instances, will need to visit the doctor's office or clinic a few days later.

In the space of one hour or so, a baby will have been born by cesarean. The precise teamwork of the doctors and nurses may seem almost nonchalant. It isn't. Years of training and a great deal of planning have gone into making the procedures appear effortless and routine. For the parents, this is a day so special they will remember it for the rest of their lives. The cesarean baby will benefit from, or be adversely affected by, both the quality of the medical, technical, surgical, and anesthetic care the mother receives, and the concern and support the parents have been accorded. There is a special beauty, a poetry, a spirituality, a closeness that comes from having a baby. For the mother, for the father, and for the baby, this has been a birthday!

THE FATHER IN THE
CESAREAN DELIVERY ROOM

Does the father* have a right to witness the birth of his baby and to support and comfort his wife when the method

*Reference to the baby's father in this chapter and elsewhere in the book is not meant to exclude or denigrate situations in which someone else of significance and comfort to the birthing woman—a

of delivery is by cesarean? Is it his right, or a privilege to be extended to a certain few under special circumstances? Is the father who observes a cesarean birth more or less likely to sue the doctor for malpractice? Won't he be a nuisance at best, and a real problem if he faints or becomes sick to his stomach? Isn't he going to get in the way? Why, indeed, should he be there at all? And who would be crazy enough to want to watch a surgical birth?

To be sure, these questions may seem ludicrous. However, there are still nonprogressive, restrictive hospitals where fathers are not as yet allowed in the delivery room for cesarean births. The fact remains that many couples wish to be together for the birth of their babies and are permitted to do so more often than not.

The feasibility of fathers in the cesarean delivery room once stirred passionate debate. In some circles, the mere suggestion caused verbal earthquakes. Some doctors were afraid that allowing fathers to be present for cesarean births would result in a greater number of malpractice suits. To date this fear has proven thoroughly without merit. It seems that the quality of care is enhanced with the father present.

In 1975, *Time* magazine carried an article entitled "Malpractice: Rx for a Crisis," which stated:

> Patients rarely sue their family physicians who often make up in compassion and concern what they lack in technical skills. But few feel reluctant to sue an aloof and unfamiliar specialist who seems to take their respect for granted and often submits a sizeable bill as well. . . .
>
> Studies have shown that the patient who is treated with compassion is likely to feel that what-

---

labor attendant or other support person—takes part in the pregnancy, labor, and delivery instead of or in addition to the father. I use the word *father* only to avoid the clumsy phrasing that would otherwise result.

ever the result, the doctor has done his best. It is the
patient who feels himself slighted—in either medical or human terms—who expresses his dissatisfaction by a lawsuit.[1]

One way of assuring a better rapport between the obstetrician and the family is to have the father attend prenatal visits.

Other influential factors in the debate over fathers witnessing cesarean births were tradition ("We just never allowed that
before"), hospital policy ("Thou shalt have no fathers in the
cesarean section room"), and bias or insecurity on the part of
the obstetrician ("I don't want any darned fathers in there
looking over my shoulder").

When there was still tremendous controversy surrounding
the question of if and when fathers would be allowed to share
in cesarean births, Dr. J. Robert McTammany, chief of obstetrics at Community General Hospital in Reading, Pennsylvania, was a pioneer among physicians who encouraged fathers
to be present. His comments about the presence of fathers
remain pertinent today. In those few areas where there are still
policy debates among hospital staffs, or if your husband is
unsure about whether he wants to be with you, Dr. McTammany's
experience may be instructive.

> We indoctrinate the couple as time permits prior to
> the surgery. If we have to do the delivery hastily
> (for example, because of fetal distress) we talk with
> the couple afterwards in more detail. In repeat
> sections, there is more time for preparation and our
> CEA [Childbirth Education Association] C-section
> group is working on a training course for repeat
> cesarean couples. We have the father present in the
> room for the induction of anesthesia—usually spinal.
> He sits off to the side of the room while everything
> gets going and then sits by his wife's left shoulder
> during the operation, where he can hold her hand

and comfort her. (If we have to use general anesthesia, I permit the father to be present anyway, since telling her about the birth and what their baby looked like is of immense value to her). He is told that he may stand up and watch as much or as little of the operation as he likes, and that he may take snapshots if he wishes. When the baby is born it is handed to the waiting delivery room nurse who does what is necessary to the child, and as soon as practicable, wraps the baby in a blanket, and gives it to the father, who then cuddles the child close and takes it to his wife to see. The three of them spend five or ten minutes together sharing, and the baby is then taken to the nursery for weighing, banding, footprinting, eye-treatment, etc. The father is told he can either go to the nursery with the baby and make phone calls, or stay with his wife for the remainder of the operation and go with her to the recovery room. Most of them stay. Later on they get the baby's weight and make phone calls.

We haven't tried nursing [breast-feeding] in the operating room yet, but often try it several hours later when the mother is back in her bed and recovered from the anesthesia. Many of the mothers go home on their third post-operative day and they do beautifully.

It is all so simple and so right. Many couples just accept it as the natural thing to do and don't understand what an unusual opportunity they have had. All are very impressed with the o.r. [operating room] routine and teamwork. In cases where there are problems—with the mother or baby—the father lends his support and sees for himself all of our efforts on behalf of the person in trouble. They feel a tremendous appreciation—almost unworthiness— for all that is done.

The same joy and excitement we have in the delivery room is, in this way, experienced in the operating room. It seems even a little more intense because there are more participants and there is great release when the outcome is successful.[2]

By being present for the birth, cesarean fathers have the opportunity to share the experience of their babies coming into the world. The father can be with his wife to coach and support her. He may even take pictures for the family album, to be cherished, admired, and passed on to the child. Afterward, both parents will be able to reminisce about the time of joy and happiness they shared as the baby was born.

If the father or another support person cannot be present for the birth (because it isn't allowed or because he doesn't want to), it's important for the hospital staff to keep him informed of the progress of both mother and baby. After all, even fathers who elect not to be there for the birth will feel frustrated, helpless, alone, and anxious.

It is important to remember how, during a ten- to fifteen-year time span, that allowing fathers to be present for cesarean deliveries was transformed from a heated controversy into a commonly accepted reality. In order to make it possible for fathers to be present at cesarean births, parents exerted consumer pressure. That meant talking with their doctors, hospital administrators, nursing staffs, etc. It also meant writing letters, joining groups of like-minded parents and professionals to lobby for change, and boycotting doctors and hospitals where parents weren't allowed to be together for the birth. Many hospitals liberalized and humanized their cesarean birth policies when confronted with economic losses: when patients switched doctors and hospitals in favor of people and places encouraging family-centered cesarean birth, the economic loss was felt. To draw more patients or a larger hospital clientele, doctors and hospital policymakers realized they had to keep up with the times and meet the demands of their potential sources of revenue.

Fathers, as has been proven time and time again, do have a right to be present for cesarean birth. More important, the entire family benefits from his presence—or that of someone close to the mother who lends love and comfort at the time of delivery.

---- 9 ----

THE RECOVERY ROOM:
A GOOD BEGINNING

The amount of time the new mother spends in the recovery room is, on the average, about three hours. It will be necessary to remain longer if there are special problems. The recovery room staff is experienced in caring for the postpartum patient, and if the maternity floor is very busy, the mother may be kept in the recovery room for longer than three hours to ensure careful, constant checking of her condition.

Some hospitals do not have an obstetrical recovery room. Newly delivered cesarean mothers may be kept in the corridor of the labor and delivery area, or in an empty labor room, or in the regular surgical recovery room, or they may be taken immediately back to their rooms on the maternity floor. If the mother has had general anesthesia, she may remember very little of this period regardless of where it takes place. Once the mother has begun to awaken and it has been ascertained that her condition is stable, she will be returned to her room. Additional medications may keep her fairly groggy for at least another eight hours after the baby is born.

If the couple has had to be separated for the baby's birth, it is often possible (and always preferable) to be reunited with the baby's father in the recovery room. (If your hospital does not have a separate maternity recovery room, some of the procedures and suggestions of this chapter may be inapplicable.) The recovery room nurses usually try to maintain a low profile for at least the first few minutes after the mother and father are together again, so that the parents can love and comfort one another, and privately rejoice in the birth of their baby. The couple may have been separated for as little as one hour, but those sixty minutes have been more significant than any other hour in their lives.

A telephone may be available in the recovery room so that the new mother and father can announce the baby's birth to relatives. Announcing the birth is exciting to the proud parents, grandparents, and older children. Talking to Mommy will reassure older children and make them feel a part of the new baby's arrival. However, some children react nonchalantly to the announcement, and this seeming lack of interest surprises and dismays some parents. It is not cause for concern or disappointment. Older children may have been prepared well in advance for the arrival of their new little sister or brother, but until they can actually see and touch the baby for themselves, they may not fully comprehend its significance. Often they say, "Oh, really?" and then launch into an account of what they have been doing.

In the excitement and stress of giving birth, many women will become sweaty or clammy, and among the first things that will take place in the recovery room is that the mother will be given a bed bath and helped to change into a clean hospital gown. This bath can be soothing and welcome, especially if it is done gently. A mouthwash or toothbrush may be offered. Vital signs (temperature, pulse, and blood pressure) will be taken every fifteen minutes or more often if necessary. The amount, consistency, and color of the vaginal discharge will be checked frequently. (This flow will last from two to six weeks.) The recovery room nurse will also check the incision and the height of the top of the uterus. This is determined by pressing on the abdomen, but sometimes the abdomen is so tender that even the most gentle pressure is excruciatingly painful. If you think the nurse is exerting too much pressure, ask her to be gentler. These examinations take just a few seconds, but they are done frequently and are very important. It takes about six weeks for the uterus to return to its normal, nonpregnant size, but there will be a dramatic, rapid shrinking immediately after delivery. A uterus that contracts surely and rapidly is less likely to become infected or to hemorrhage.

To help stimulate contraction of the uterus, Pitocin may be added to the intravenous solution. Pitocin (sometimes called "Pit") is the same substance that is used to stimulate or induce labor. As the uterus contracts of its own accord, and/or with the help of Pitocin, the mother may experience contractions like those of labor. The intensity of these contractions varies from woman to woman and from one pregnancy to another. Should the contractions become painful at any time, or should you feel as though you are having one continuous, uninterrupted contraction, be sure to tell the nurse. Mild cramping at intervals is to be expected. Continual pain is not. The Pitocin may be flowing too rapidly from the IV. The nurse will be able to slow down the IV or discontinue the Pitocin altogether (with your doctor's permission) or give additional pain medication if necessary. A few mild cramps can be managed with pain medication and/or slow, controlled relaxation breathing. It is thought that postpartum contractions may be more intense with second and subsequent pregnancies, although the reasons are still the subject of medical study. The cesarean mother should remember that she has had a baby and that her body must make adjustments to compensate for the swift change from mother-to-be to mother-in-fact. (Incidentally, the Pitocin may be continued for at least a few hours after the mother has been returned to her room, so the problem of intense afterbirth contractions, if it is to occur, may not surface until then.)

Soon after she has been taken to the recovery room, the

mother's legs will regain sensation if she has had spinal anesthesia. Sometimes the legs begin to tingle or feel the way legs do when they have fallen asleep. The sensation usually begins at the toes and progresses upward. The nurse will ask the mother to move her legs. At first, the mother's brain may send the command but receive no response. Gradually motor control will return. This regaining of sensation has been described by different mothers as being "weird," "prickly," and "oddly uncomfortable"—but never painful.

In the recovery room, one or more injections may be given to alleviate pain. These may make the mother sleepy, groggy, or drowsy. At this time, the excitement of the day's events combined with the physical strain of the cesarean delivery may make the mother feel "spaced out" or "out of it completely." Some mothers are so happy and high that sleep is out of the question. They chat with the baby's father and talk the nurses' ears off. The mother who does feel sleepy is encouraged to give in to that feeling. If the father is there, he will certainly understand that this rest is beneficial.

The amount of discomfort experienced in the recovery room (and during the remainder of the hospital stay) varies from woman to woman, and even from delivery to delivery. Some mothers feel little or no discomfort, while others report that they were totally miserable and in severe pain. How much pain you experience should *not* be considered a negative reflection on your coping abilities. If at any time you feel uncomfortable or unable to cope effectively, inform the nurses immediately. Most obstetricians make only brief rounds, so it is the nurses on whom you must depend. They, in turn, will communicate any special problems requiring immediate attention to your obstetrician or anesthesiologist.

As a general rule throughout the hospital stay, it is a good idea to take pain medication before discomfort becomes severe. This way the medication will work more effectively and sooner. Playing Superwoman or trying to tough it out without any medication at all is not necessary, nor even especially helpful.

You have had a baby and an operation. A cesarean delivery is not an endurance test. Feeling uncomfortable does not mean that you are a weakling or a failure. Knowing what to expect and how to cope effectively with any situation will help to make your recuperative period easier.

Headaches, as the direct result of spinal anesthesia, will occur within a few hours or days of delivery *if* they are to happen at all. (Anesthesia will not be the cause of headaches that occur months or years after delivery.) You may experience shoulder pain, caused by air having collected under the diaphragm as a result of surgery. Tell the doctor or nurse if you have either a headache or shoulder pain, or both. They are not major problems but can be aggravating, especially in conjunction with the other physical debilities that may occur as the result of just having delivered a baby by cesarean. Thanks to new techniques, headaches from anesthesia are less frequent nowadays.

Both the bladder catheter and the IV will remain in place for a varying number of hours. How soon either or both are removed depends on the doctor's orders and the mother's condition. Some doctors prefer to have them kept in place for a day or two.

Equally as important as the physical care the mother receives in the recovery room is the fulfillment of her need to begin the "mothering" processes. For healthy, normal mothering patterns to flourish and grow, the mother and her baby must be reunited as soon as possible. While the anesthesia is still partially in effect, the mother should be quite comfortable physically. Coupled with the elation of giving birth, the first hour or two in the recovery room is a superb time for mother and father to become acquainted with their baby, and for the mother to initiate breast-feeding. Even if she does not breastfeed, early, close physical contact will promote the maternal-infant bonding processes and reassure mother, father, and baby. (See Chapter 12.)

What will make the mother most happy in the recovery

room is having her baby with her. She may have been able to kiss and touch her new baby in the delivery room, but holding her baby in her arms is an experience without equal. Unless the baby is truly endangered and cannot be taken from the special care nursery, both mother and baby will benefit from this early, close contact. The baby will be reassured by her mother's heartbeat, a sound that has been familiar to her during the entire gestation process. The mother will be able to examine her baby closely and to see for herself that the child is well. No matter what anyone else tells her about her baby's perfection, nothing can replace her own inspection.

The mother will need help holding and feeding her baby. The nurse or baby's father can make the mother comfortable by helping her to turn on her side, propping pillows under her back, adjusting the bed for comfort, and helping her to loosen her hospital gown so that her baby can have skin-to-skin contact and access to her mother's breast. The baby's father may lift the baby from her crib and place her in the mother's arms. This contact will help to promote his sense of closeness to the baby.

Newborn babies are often "barracudas" and take to sucking with vigor. Sometimes, however, instead of being a go-getter, the baby is sleepy and won't nurse right away. New mothers need to know that they are doing a good job of caring for their babies. Snuggling together, with the nurse and baby's father nearby to lend assurance, will promote the mother's sense of security.

When the mother has finished nursing on one breast, the baby's father can burp the baby, place her in her crib, and then rearrange the pillows and help the mother turn onto her other side for feeding. There should always be a pillow on the mother's lap to splint the incision and take the weight of the baby's body off this very tender area.

The benefits of nursing the baby within a short time after birth are numerous. As noted earlier, some cesarean mothers may nurse their babies while still on the delivery table. The advantages of early touching and nursing include mother-baby skin contact, the reassurance of the mother's heartbeat to the newborn, and the immunities provided by colostrum (the first milk secreted). Numerous studies have shown that face-to-face contact of mother and father with the baby and tactile stimulation of the newborn—especially the cesarean newborn— are vital. If you feel inexpert at first, that is perfectly natural.

Some newborns have difficulty maintaining a stable body temperature at first. The warmth of the mother's (or father's) body and arms are the best baby-warmer unit ever devised. You may be concerned as parents that you won't know how to hold the baby properly, that you won't know what to do for or with her. Even if you have a ten pounder, your baby will look so helpless, so tiny, so fragile. She isn't as delicate as she looks.

New cesarean mothers also need coddling and care right after birth. You may be exhausted as a result of having had a cesarean and then from holding the baby and celebrating the birth. While the baby is with you, however, you may be so enthralled and ecstatic that you forget all about yourself—at least for the time being. When (and if) the baby is taken to the nursery or settles down in her crib beside you for a nap, you may welcome this opportunity to fall blissfully asleep. The first contact with your baby should be as long as possible. But even if you and your baby are together only a few minutes, this is a very important time.

If the baby cannot be brought to you in the recovery room (either because of an outdated hospital policy or because your baby must remain in a special care nursery so that her condition can be monitored, the amount of oxygen she receives regulated, and the temperature and humidity controlled), the baby's father or a special friend or relative appointed by you may wish to take some Polaroid pictures of the baby at frequent intervals to show to you. A member of the hospital staff could also do this if you're alone.

Some hospitals have Polaroid cameras on the maternity floor for use by parents. It is better to bring your own (and lots of film) since not all hospitals have cameras. These photographs can bring immediate reassurance to the mother and will later be treasured by the parents—even if they are a little disappointed at first at the appearance of their baby. Newborns are often wrinkly, scrunched up, and less than glamorous. Bringing your own instant camera will also enable you to take lots of pictures for the grandparents and older children. The new mother who cannot be with her baby for hours (or, in a few cases, days) will want to have pictures taken frequently because the newborn baby changes rapidly—sometimes even from one hour to the next.

Good communications between the nursery staff and the recovery room nurses is essential at all times—but particularly if inflexible hospital policy dictates that the mother cannot have anyone with her in the recovery room. Even when the baby's father is with the mother, and the baby is to be brought to her, there may be a short observation period varying from a few minutes to a few hours, depending on hospital policy, the availability of a pediatrician or special nurse to give the go-ahead, and/or the baby's temperature. Usually there is a drop in the baby's temperature immediately after birth. Before the baby can be brought to the mother, her temperature must rise to normal and remain stable. During this time, the mother may ask and re-ask for frequent reports on the baby's condition. The reporter may become a bit exasperated, but until the mother can see for herself, this constant reiteration is vitally important to her.

ABDOMINAL TIGHTENING EXERCISE TO REDUCE GAS DISCOMFORT

Although gas pains do not usually occur until several days after delivery, one hour after the baby's birth is the time to begin using this technique to help reduce (and in some cases, eliminate) what many mothers call "the *worst* aspect of having a cesarean"—gas. After a cesarean, the condition is *never* "only gas." It is GAS and it can hurt!

Gas forms because the intestines have temporarily stopped working efficiently due to the fact that (1) the mother has had anesthesia and a host of other medications; (2) the intestines have been exposed to air and handled during the operation; and (3) the mother is unable to move about freely as is necessary to help stimulate normal intestinal action. Not every cesarean mother gets a painful bout of gas. For those who do, the suffering it produces varies from mild to severe. For maximum effect, begin this abdominal tightening exercise within one hour after delivery, and do it four or five times an hour *every* hour that you are awake, for at least five days. Although this technique can be used by anyone who has undergone abdominal surgery, an added bonus for the cesarean mother is that it will make it easier for her to move about comfortably and to care for her baby during the first few postpartum days. Here is the exercise recommended by Valmai Elkins of Montreal, a Registered Physical Therapist.

First, place both hands over your incision to form a splint. If you like, place a small pillow directly over your abdomen for further support, and then join both hands together on top of the pillow, just over the incision. Take a deep "welcoming" breath in and then let it all out. Take another deep breath and hold it to the slow count of five. Holding to the count of ten is better if you can manage it but don't push yourself too hard, at least the first few times you try. When you have finished counting, let the breath out, and take a final deep "parting" breath in and let it out. Elizabeth Noble, R.P.T., author of *Essential Exercises for the Childbearing Years,* teaches another variation of this in her book. Her method advocates pushing the abdomen out, rather than holding it in. Both ways are effective. The important thing to remember with the Elkins technique is that when you're holding the breath in, really pull in your gut as tightly as you can. When exhaling to complete the exercise, really push your abdomen out as far as it will go. A good check to determine if you're doing this effectively and properly is to have someone else place a hand on your abdomen to make sure you're really pulling it in on the inhale while you count to five, and pushing it out as you're finishing up with an exhale. (If you have clamps instead of sutures, place both hands beside the clamps. It's not really necessary, but it will make you feel more secure.)

The hospital where you deliver may already use this technique, and one of the recovery room nurses may remind you to begin abdominal tightening as a matter of postoperative routine. If not, ask your husband to put this on his checklist of things to do. The first few times you try this technique it may be uncomfortable. It becomes easier each time. Also, you may be afraid to do it for fear the incision may come apart. That won't happen. Abdominal tightening is important to help make your recovery smoother and more comfortable.

A Good Beginning. In the recovery room you may feel a combination of physical sensations, euphoria, triumph, jubilation, fatigue, and relief. A good recovery room experience, like a good delivery, will be a positive beginning for you as a family. Uniting parents and baby in the recovery room is a way of making the cesarean delivery a family-centered event and will see you off to a good relationship with your baby, and your baby with you.

The long wait is over. The baby is healthy, beautiful, and yours for keeps. Hallelujah! Now it is time to rejoice, relax, and begin to recover.

THE POSTPARTUM
HOSPITAL STAY

To paraphrase Reeva Rubin, professor and director of the Graduate Program in Maternity Nursing at the University of Pittsburgh, it's pretty hard to feel maternal when your mouth tastes unpleasant and your back feels like a twisted lead pipe. Cesarean mothers are handicapped by a lack of mobility and by physical discomfort, which sometimes makes it difficult for them to establish their roles as caretaker and nurturer in the first few days and weeks after birth. The cesarean mother needs rest, relaxation, and support. In a word: she, too, needs coddling.

The hospital stay will be about three to five days. Some women are released after two or three days, most stay five, and a few require a week or more. Try not to be in a hurry to get home. An extra day or two in the hospital may be beneficial, especially if there is an older child or children at home, and/or you do not have someone there to help you out.

A very few women breeze through the recovery period. Their incisions cause only minor concern. Nothing bothers them—neither their own bodies nor the needs of the newborn. They are ecstatic. Within a few days of delivery, they are happy and home. Within weeks, they may be doing all the things they normally did before the baby was born and may even tackle tasks such as wallpapering the baby's room, which other mothers cannot do for months.

At the other end of the spectrum are women who, through no fault of their own, have complications. Their incisions may become infected; they may develop a high fever or hemorrhaging may occur; a totally unrelated illness such as the flu or a cold strikes them; or they may suffer a reaction to one of the drugs administered. No matter how positive their attitudes, their bodies are truly debilitated. Complications can happen.

There is a tiny group of mothers who, like characters in soap operas, use their birthing experiences as convenient pegs on which to hang *all* their troubles. From the moment they awaken from anesthesia and for years afterward, their "horrible, just *horrible*" operation is a favorite topic. Everything that happens to them from then on is blamed on their "sections." (These women do not give birth by cesarean, they have Sections, with a capital "S".)

The vast majority of cesarean mothers fall somewhere in the middle of the spectrum. They, too, must talk about and relive their experiences. It is natural and healthy. Talking about what happened will enable them to finalize the experience. These women are delighted to be mothers, but their bodies are not as cooperative as their minds. They cannot move freely. Walking, sneezing, laughing, and coughing become "unnatural" and painful. Their bodies need time to repair themselves, and their babies want to snuggle, nurse, and be loved at the same time. What can be done to help smooth over the first few postpartum days? There are steps the mother, father, and hospital staff can take that will have a very positive effect on the way the parents relate to the baby and will help to transform the "container of pain" into a comfortable, loving mother.

The first twenty-four hours or so after delivery will probably be fairly hazy. Fatigue, pain medication, and a sense of relief and accomplishment make the new mother very tired. You may remember very little of what happens the first day. Relax and take it easy. Your body will dictate how much or how little you should do. You have just given birth and deserve to think only of yourself—for a few hours, at least. If you force yourself too much, you will not make a very cheerful mother when the baby is brought to you. If you want to have full rooming-in, you may prefer to initiate it after you've had a day or two in which to regain your strength.

It is essential to continue the abdominal tightening exercise (see page 140). If you forgot to begin in the recovery room, it is not too late, although maximum benefit may be reduced. Not all hospitals are as yet familiar with this exercise, and you may be asked what you're doing and why.

Both to relieve gas and to speed the recuperative period, it is best to turn as often and as frequently as possible while you are still confined to bed. It is probably going to hurt at first. Relaxation breathing techniques will help those first few times you shift your position. It gets easier each time.

Check your position in bed several times a day. As the day progresses, you may end up "scrunched up" at the foot of the bed. Try to remember to keep yourself in a lying down flat or sitting position.

Within twenty-four hours of delivery, you will take your first trip out of bed. Even if you are feeling on top of the world, the first trip should not be undertaken unless there is a nurse in the room. You will need help in case you get dizzy or feel faint. Just the effort of sitting up the first time may make you feel dizzy. The baby's father or your support person may be present at this time, but other visitors should not be. Getting out of bed and walking to a chair will require a great deal of effort. Also, the effort may possibly cause a sudden, profuse gush of vaginal discharge, which you may find embarrassing if there are other people in the room.

The most outstanding sensation every new cesarean mother has as she tries to sit up, swing her legs over the side of the bed, and stand is a pulling or tugging in the area around the incision. In fact, if this is your first cesarean, this feeling may come as an unpleasant shock. You may think your incision is going to split apart and the entire contents of your insides tumble out onto the floor. The incision will not come apart, but it is a feeling experienced by almost every cesarean mother. To compensate for this sensation, which may be experienced as a minor feeling of discomfort or as a searing pain, you will be inclined to bend from the waist, to stoop, and to do what is called the "cesarean shuffle." Don't. The cesarean shuffle is highly discouraged, even though it may take a great deal of effort to stand straight and tall. Remember to walk like a high-fashion model the first and every time that you walk. How bad it can hurt to stand and walk should not be underestimated. It may hurt like the blue blazes. Fortunately, it gets easier each time. The more you move about, the earlier you do so, and the straighter you stand, the sooner you will be able to move gracefully and effortlessly.

The first walk (which some mothers liken to the "incredible journey" in *Pilgrim's Progress*) can be accomplished even if the IV and catheter are still in place. It may seem to take forever just to walk from the bed to a chair a few feet away.

What and when you are allowed to eat depends on your doctor's preferences and your condition. The IV may be kept running for several days. Through the IV you will receive water, glucose or dextrose (sugar), saline (salt), and/or medication. You may be allowed only room-temperature water and juices for days, while another cesarean mother, who delivered the same time you did, may be served dinner that evening. She probably has another doctor. The major reason for conservatism with regard to diet is the belief that limiting the diet may reduce the discomforts of gas and constipation. However, liberalized postoperative orders that allow for food shortly after delivery are becoming more widely advocated. Insist upon discussing this with your doctor during pregnancy and include it in your "Birth Requests" list.

Being very, very thirsty after having a baby is not uncommon. Water and/or ice chips are welcome thirst-quenchers. From water, you may progress to broth, juices, mineral water and soda (cola, ginger ale, etc.)—although it is advisable to sip carbonated beverages through a straw after some of the bubbles have dissipated. Gelatin will probably be the first food you will be allowed to eat. After all those liquids, the first few dishes are very tasty, but then you may notice that breakfast, lunch, and dinner all bear a disheartening resemblance: gelatin or custard, clear broth, and tea. That is fine—for a while. After what seems like an eternity of broth, tea, and gelatin, you may become so hungry that you would do anything to have some real food. When the nurse walks into your room carrying still another tray of custard and broth, your reaction may be to cry or get angry.

It can be demoralizing to be forbidden "real" food for a period of days. Cesarean mothers and their obstetricians are often able to compromise. Herb teas, yogurt, mashed potatoes, creamed soups and vegetables, roast turkey and chicken, broiled fish, rice cereal, or farina may be foods the doctor will allow. They will satisfy the mother's hunger, her body's need for nutrition, and concurrently lift her morale without adding undue strain on her digestive system.

If you really must have something solid to eat, and your doctor forbids it for longer than you think necessary, you could cheat. You could sneak a few cookies, a candy bar, or something forbidden. If you do, you'll suffer for it. Such foods are certain to cause gas pains and may lead to constipation. Try to be reasonable and intelligent in making a decision like that and choose easily digested, nutritious foods.

The subject of adequate, proper nutrition following surgery is just now being reevaluated by the medical profession. Some doctors are well acquainted with the intense needs of the postsurgical patient for vitamins, minerals, and trace elements. If is known that they are greatly depleted during physical trauma. Some of these elements can be stored in the body and released into the system gradually. Others must be replenished daily. If you are concerned about the need for adequate nutrition, you should discuss it with your obstetrician, preferably during a prenatal visit. If your doctor prefers a truly conservative diet, you may request vitamin tablets to give a much-needed boost during those first few days when you are restricted as to what you may eat and drink.

Pain medication will be offered for at least two or three days and probably longer. At first it will be given as an injection and later as pills. It is true that some of this medication will go through the mother's milk and into the baby. The amount passed on to the baby is minimal, and the mother may find it difficult indeed to be really "maternal" if she is in pain. Pain may vary from mild discomfort to a temporarily excruciating sensation. There are times when you will want to take the medication offered—and may even find it difficult to wait for the next dose. At other times, your need may not be as great. You'll discover how often you need to have medication. Remember, too, that the dosage is usually reduced gradually. If you need pain medication while in the hospital, take it. You won't become a drug addict in a few short days, nor will your baby be adversely affected by it. If you don't need it, you have the right to refuse it. On the other hand, don't wait until you are so uncomfortable you can hardly see straight before asking for it. It won't work as effectively then.

Cesarean mothers should not compare their progress (nor be compared by others) with the progress of a vaginally delivering mother, or in fact, with that of another cesarean mother. How quickly and easily one recuperates varies from woman to woman and even from one pregnancy to the next. The cesarean mother has special considerations and handicaps that must be taken into account.

One excellent innovation some hospitals have introduced is the use of color-coded tags on the cribs of all babies delivered by cesarean. It is often impossible for nurses to remember which mothers had cesareans if there are many mothers on the maternity floor. These tags remind them that this mother and baby need extra time and attention. Tags on cribs automatically alert nurses to the fact that they will have to help the mother achieve a comfortable position for feeding (a pillow placed on the abdomen, and one or two under her back) and place the baby in the mother's arms before leaving the room. The nurse will also have to return to the mother's room within a few minutes to help her burp the baby and change sides for feedings. If the nurse does not return, the intercom or buzzer should be used—that's what they're there for.

Sometimes cesarean mothers are placed in rooms together and preferably in rooms closest to the nursery. Although it is not always possible, because of a "baby boom" or lack of beds, being with others who have shared a similar experience serves many useful purposes. For one thing, the cesarean mother won't be depressed when her roommate bounces out of bed minutes or hours after a vaginal delivery, while she is still having trouble getting to and from the bathroom two, three, or four days after delivery. Cesarean mothers will be able to share their experiences and trade tips on how to deal with everything from the incision to the baby. Placing cesarean mothers in rooms closest to the nursery makes the walk less trying and tiring and will be especially appreciated those first few post-partum days. Many hospitals now have electric beds for all their patients. But when there are only a few available, it is thoughtful (and necessary) to save them for cesarean mothers. Being able to press a button to elevate her head or knees, or lower the bed so she can get out without having to call a nurse, is a small but important consideration, which also frees the nursing staff to do other things.

During the postpartum stay, the nursing staff or a special clinician may spend some time with cesarean mothers so they can talk about their experiences, ask questions, and relieve themselves of any psychological stress if they wish. If the mother was traumatized by the event, being able to talk about it will help her to sort out and work through any problems she may have. Negative experiences sometimes assume proportions far in excess of reality. If cesarean mothers are not afforded the benefits of someone to talk with, their impressions of the experience may become increasingly more bitter and horrifying.

Support groups, composed primarily of cesarean parents, are growing in number. Through these organizations, postpartum cesarean mothers are sometimes visited in the hospital. Although the woman who comes to visit will not be able to give medical advice (she does not need to—many doctors and nurses are on hand to fill this need), she will be able to listen and to talk with the mother about her own experiences and may help the new mother to cope with the myriad problems. It is important to erase the negative tapes playing in the minds of cesarean mothers, particularly those whose birth experiences have been anything but ideal. Emoting about the experience, in the company of someone who is empathetic and skilled at peer counseling, will benefit the new cesarean parent. What is needed and what is gained is an understanding of the emotional and physical aspects of the event from someone who has undergone a similar experience. If the cesarean mother feels isolated, frustrated or has questions, this informal chat may be just the thing needed to overcome these feelings.

During the first few days after delivery, the new mother's body will change dramatically. After months of feeling like an overweight hippopotamus, the reduction in waist size is welcome. Like any new mother, cesarean women must wear those giant sanitary pads (euphemistically called "mouse mattresses"). Unless the hospital provides the kind of pads that have adhesive backing, a sanitary belt must be worn. Occasionally, the clasps on the belt bite into the skin. Using safety pins rather than a belt may be more comfortable. Tampons should not be used. The lochia (vaginal discharge and bleeding), which continues for two to six weeks after delivery, is a good external indicator should internal problems arise. At any time during the postpartum period, if the amount of flow increases, or if there are clots or an unusually foul smell, you should tell your doctor. (If you are at home, an increased flow usually means you are doing too much. Go to bed at once, prop your feet up, and let the dust and disorder accumulate.) Like women who deliver vaginally, it will be necessary for the cesarean mother to cleanse the perineal area each time she urinates, for as long as the bleeding and discharge continue. This cleansing will reduce the chance of infection. Always wipe from front to back. (The anal and vaginal openings are very close together, so wiping from back to front may cause infection.)

In the hospital, cotton gowns are preferable to synthetic ones. Nylon and rayon cling and become easily twisted. Cotton gowns are also cooler. Hospitals are known to be overheated and the body of the new mother, which is going through a readjustment, may cause her to perspire profusely or have hot flashes. Finding pretty cotton gowns that open in the front—an important consideration for mothers who nurse their babies—is becoming easier. If you can't find anything suitable in the sleepwear department, try substituting at-home wear instead.

While you are in the hospital, try to get as much rest as possible. Hospital routine, which includes frequent checks on vital signs, visits from the doctor, messengers bringing flowers and mail, bed baths or showers, room cleaning, changing the linen, and bringing medication, may inhibit rather than promote rest. With all the necessary routines of the hospital, many women find that each time they doze off, someone else comes into the room. Closing the door and posting a No Visitors or Do Not Disturb sign helps . . . sometimes. With a sign on the door, most people will at least knock. The mother may begin to feel that she will never get enough rest. She will, but it will take some time. Later on at home, she and baby can settle into their own beds, take the phone off the hook, enforce a No Visitors rule, and delegate the housework to the father, grandmother, or friend.

Coughing, laughing, and sneeezing may rekindle your fears about rupturing the incision. Because of surgery, medications, and confinement to bed (for at least twelve hours), you may find the desire to cough greater at this time. In an effort to guard the incision, you may try to suppress your cough. Don't. Instead, splint the incision with your hands and/or a pillow, then take a deep breath in, let it out, take another deep breath, and cough! Holding the cough back only makes matters worse. Coughing also promotes functioning of the lungs at full capacity again.

Some hospitals provide binders for cesarean mothers. A binder is a wide elastic belt that fits around the abdomen and is used for support. It may lessen the discomfort initially, but it has disadvantages. The binder can become a crutch and give you a false sense of security. It will also allow your abdominal muscles to relax rather than to tone and strengthen themselves. Weakened muscles will cause more discomfort in the long run and require a longer period for you to shape up and regain your figure. If it's absolutely necessary, use a binder, but do so judiciously. To promote better circulation, some doctors order support stockings or socks.

An annoyance following cesarean childbirth is itching of the incision. In fact, some women report that just thinking about the birth or hearing the word "cesarean" causes the scar to itch even months later. If itching is a problem, it may be helpful to scratch *another* part of your body. It just isn't polite to scratch the incision in some instances, especially if the incision is the lower segment type. Once the scar heals, vitamin E or pure aloe vera may also relieve the itchiness. You can still wear a two-piece bathing suit or bikini, but you should block the sun's rays from the incision for about six months after delivery.

How well the scar heals depends primarily upon the mother's skin type. Standing straight and tall from the first time out of bed helps the skin incision to heal more neatly, too. Some skin types produce a raised shiny red scar, called a keloid, no matter how much care is taken. Sometimes the incision will fade almost totally, so that after a year or so, it is almost indiscernible. One advantage to the lower segment "bikini cut" is that after the pubic hair grows in, it becomes almost totally covered by the hair. One woman, who had planned an at-home delivery but who had to have a cesarean because the baby was breech and very large, said, "I never felt at all unattractive, even when the scar was fresh. It was like a merit badge. That's the way my beautiful baby decided to come into the world, so it didn't bother me at all, ever." Hers is a very positive attitude. There are other women who feel mutilated by the scar. Classical incisions are more likely to cause this type of resentment. The new mother may feel that she has become less attractive, and perhaps less sexually appealing to her mate. She may also worry that she will be unable to wear a bikini again. Nonsense. To be sure, the scar may cause some hesitation the first summer season, but it should not keep a woman out of a bikini if she has the figure for one anyway. Most people don't notice the scar at all, although the mother may think it is glaring.

There will also be "The Day the Milk Came In," usually about the third postpartum day. Women with small breasts will look like voluptuous models. One's breast size is unrelated to one's ability to provide adequate milk to one's baby. Your milk is nature's way of providing the perfect food for your baby. A hot-water bottle or heating pad, a hot shower, or wearing a bra for support—and patience—will help to relieve any temporary discomfort caused by engorgement of the breasts. Nursing the baby will bring the greatest relief.

About the third day after delivery, you may get a case of the blues. The new mother may find herself in tears for no obvious reason, or for a trivial one. Perhaps the baby starts to cry when the mother has just settled down for a nap. Being hungry may trigger the tears. The mother may be starving for real food. And there it is again: a tray full of gelatin, tea, and broth. The mother may hold back the tears (if she can) until the nurse leaves the room, and then the floodgates open. If the mother is feeling physically uncomfortable, her depression may be magnified.

No matter what triggers her depression, the result is the same: the mother feels sad and miserable, or helpless and guilty. She *should* be happy (or so she tells herself) because everything is going well. The baby is healthy, beautiful, and hers at last. In a few days, she'll be going home. Normally the mother is very independent. Now she must rely very heavily upon others to do things for her. So she cries. And woe to the father who comes to the hospital late on this day! His tardiness, however unintentional, is bound to make the mother feel even more sad and lonely. An understanding, loving father will accept the blues with equanimity, and do everything he can to comfort his wife.

Although postpartum depression is usually no better or worse than for vaginally delivering mothers, there is one instance in which postpartum depression may be greater for the cesarean mother. The mother who anticipated a vaginal delivery may be devastated by the unexpected turn of events. She had high expectations and had read or heard glowing accounts of the wonders and beauties of birth. She may have gone to childbirth classes and diligently practiced the breathing exercises. She feels cheated and unhappy. The mother who has had a surprise cesarean may feel that her femininity has been undermined. She may think she has failed herself, her husband, her baby, perhaps even her instructor. She may resent her body for having let her down, her baby for complicating matters, the hospital staff for not supporting her sufficiently or for giving her too much or too little medication. She thinks she's failed the test.

After a cesarean delivery, being unable to move effortlessly and being tired may also cause negative feelings, which may be compounded by seeing roommates who delivered vaginally at midnight have a complete breakfast and walk down to the nursery at 7 A.M. The cesarean mother may not articulate her negative feelings, if she has them, or even acknowledge them. She may seem uncommunicative or difficult to deal with, but she needs extra support and encouragement from her mate and the hospital staff.

Whatever the reason, postpartum depression can be very real and very traumatic. It may not surface until weeks later. It may be worse for the woman who delivers in the winter, when inclement weather traps her in the house for days at a time. Postpartum depression may not happen at all.

The physical stress of surgery, the demands of the newborn, the needs of the father and older children, the hormonal changes of going from pregnancy to nonpregnancy, singly or in combination, may create problems that range from mild blues to severe anxiety or depression. Fatigue, from trying to accomplish too much too soon, may increase the problem. The cesarean mother should give her body a chance to heal and remember that recovery, physical and emotional, will come. It may take a few days or even weeks for full physical recovery and a return to emotional balance, but it will happen. Women who are well-adjusted and delighted to be mothers can expect at least one or two rocky days when nothing seems to go right. The father's support, his participation in the mother's and baby's care, and a nursing staff that appreciates the special status of the cesarean mother will enable her to see things in a more positive perspective.

Rooming-in is possible for cesarean mothers, despite rumors to the contrary. You may want to modify the plan to partial rooming-in for the first few days so that the baby is with you only for short periods, rather than all day and all night. No matter how good the mother feels, she will tire quickly. She should not feel guilty if she wants to send the baby back to the nursery so that she can relax and nap. She will be a better mother if she is rested and comfortable. The quality of time spent with the baby is far superior to the quantity.

Three things that will speed recovery and allow cesarean mothers to take an active part in the care and feeding of their newborns are a supportive hospital staff, flexible policy, and Family-Centered Maternity Care. FCMC is, in essence, the philosophy of regarding the mother, father, and baby as a unit. To this end, fathers are encouraged to spend as much time as they like at the hospital and to take an active role in caring for the mother and baby. Even if this baby is the couple's second, third, or fourth, the parents will want to familiarize themselves with her unique personality, her unique rhythms, preferences, and eccentricities before going home, where there may be other children who need tending and less time to spend with each child individually. The father and mother who see their baby born, who hold her within minutes of birth, and who share the joys and responsibilities of parenting are apt to be better parents, able to relate to their baby in a very special way.

Separation of the family at the time of birth and during the hospital stay is a fairly recent innovation. Until early in this century, women gave birth at home. Slowly hospitals gained favor, and "germs" became the byword and testament of the medical profession. Mothers—and *especially* fathers—became harbingers of contamination. Babies were placed in sterile nurseries (which Ashley Montague says are so named because nursing—that is, breast-feeding—is the only thing that doesn't take place there) and brought to their mothers every four hours for feeding: no more, no less. The babies' fussiness and colic were blamed on mothers, rather than on the well-intentioned but inhumane hospital routine. Visiting hours for fathers were limited to an hour or two per day.

It is appalling to think that practices introduced in the 1920s should still be in effect in the '80s. In an effort to be "modern," some hospitals have missed the point of what is best for the mother, father, and baby. The infant has come from a comfortable, warm, dark environment into the brightly lit nursery, with its clear plastic cribs and prepackaged formulas. Blankets, shirts, and diapers, no matter how well-washed and fabric-softened, must scratch the newborn's tender flesh. Nurses, however sweet, loving, and dedicated, cannot replace the mother's arms and the familiar sound of her heartbeat and voice.

Fortunately, many hospitals are now moving toward Family-Centered Maternity Care. (A hospital with Family-Centered Maternity Care may not describe its program with those exact words even though its program incorporates the elements of FCMC.) FCMC policies include liberal visiting hours (often hospitals permit fathers to visit from 6 or 7 A.M. to 11 P.M.) or round-the-clock visitation to accommodate fathers with work schedules that don't permit them to come to the hospital during the day. In deference to germs, the father is usually required to wear a hospital gown and sometimes a mask when the baby is in the mother's room. If the baby is not already in the room when he arrives, the father may go to the nursery for her. He can help make the mother comfortable for feedings, burp the baby, change diapers, or hold the child in his arms, study her features, count her fingers and toes, and do all the things fathers are supposed to and want to do.

Given the motivation and opportunity, the father is also a good coach who can remind the mother to do her abdominal tightening exercises, to get out of bed and stand straight. He can lend an arm as she walks, brush her hair, help her get into the shower, stand by in case she becomes dizzy and needs help, rub her back, mop her brow, bring water and drinks, answer the phone, or run errands. These may seem like menial tasks, but the mother will very much appreciate them. These "little" things may tip the balance between a speedy recovery and one that is just mediocre. While many of these tasks can be accomplished by a nurse, the T.L.C. that only the father can give is what makes the difference.

Bath demonstrations, breast-feeding classes, and infant care programs are often open to fathers as well as mothers. These programs are usually offered several times a week (sometimes daily) but some hospitals do not have them. They are excellent ways of supporting and reassuring parents for taking care of baby at home.

Family-Centered Maternity Care allows older children to visit Mommy in the hospital. Little ones are eager to reassure themselves that Mommy is all right, and they want to see their new little brother or sister. What used to be a lump in the mother's abdomen has become a little person who caused Mommy to go to the hospital. Is Mommy okay? What does the new baby look like? The "stranger" in the hospital becomes more of a reality and less of a threat when glimpsed first hand. Some parents fear that older children will cry and be sad when the time comes for them to leave Mommy and baby in the hospital. It is probably better that older children see their mother and cry (if they are going to) than not to see her at all. More often than not, the older children will not cry when they leave. Usually it is the mothers who do! A child's sense of time is not as well-developed as an adult's. If the children are with Grandma or a friend, they'll probably be quite happy to leave Mommy to go home to watch a favorite television program or have ice cream as a special treat. A long-range plus to sibling visiting is that most youngsters never visit hospitals unless they are admitted for illness or injury. Coming to the hospital at a time of happiness will make the hospital a less threatening place.

This new awareness of the special, different needs of cesarean families on the part of hospital staffs makes the difference between competent care and excellent, first-rate care. For the parents, this new understanding has special bonuses: they are delighted to discover that they are having better birth experiences and easier, more positive postpartum periods.

Going home is eagerly awaited. The new mother counts the

days until she will be able to sleep in her own bed again, eat anything she wants to, and set up life with the new baby without the well-intentioned interruptions of hospital routines and schedules. If this is the parents' first baby, they may also feel the responsibilities of parenthood quite heavily. The new baby is so tiny, so helpless, and so dependent on the mother and father for nourishment and love. How can they possibly do the right things? Where do they go from here?

THE "FOURTH" TRIMESTER

When the day for going home arrives, the mother, for the first time in months, is able to don a pair of jeans or slacks, or a dress of *approximately* the size she used to wear before pregnancy enveloped her. (The word "approximately" is intentional. It comes as a very discouraging blow to some mothers to learn that they still have to wear something looser than normal in order to allow for the increase in breast size and the still-flabby belly.) The baby is dressed in a brand new outfit, specially selected for going home. The father arrives at the hospital early to help get the family organized and to sign the appropriate papers. If there is a delay (either because the bill has not been computed or because there is no one available to escort the mother and baby to the car), the parents become jittery.

At last all is ready. The mother and father are safely seatbelted, and the baby is placed in a car seat designed for safety. It is never too early to ensure the baby's well-being in the car. Minor accidents can have disastrous consequences for the baby held in the mother's lap. Seat belts and baby car seats are now mandatory in many states—and should be mandatory for your family.

Even if the ride home is short, the mother may be exhausted by the time they arrive. The excitement of going home, dressing herself and the baby, and riding in the car may wear her out. At home, older children or proud grandparents may be waiting. The mother finds that she is overjoyed to greet her family and that the most comfortable spot for her is in her own bed. Everything around her is familiar and reassuring. She and the baby settle down while the father and grandparents make lunch, play with older children, and cuddle the new baby. There is something very special and magical about a new baby. Every friend and relative within miles wants to get a close look as soon as possible. Their visits are often both welcome and taxing. At last the phone stops ringing, and the family settles down into a nice, happy routine—or so it is assumed.

If the baby is a first child, most parents envision this time of adjusting from couple to family in much the way it is pictured on television and in magazine advertisements. The mother, father, and baby are always smiling. The baby is immaculately dressed, and the mother, beautifully coiffed and wearing a white designer gown, sits in a bentwood rocking chair. All is lovely, peaceful, and elegant. This is pure fantasy.

Then reality strikes. If your baby's gown was ever immaculate, you will learn that it does not remain so for long. Real babies will spit up all over even designer creations, and the most highly touted diapers, either from the diaper service or disposable, will sometimes leak. The new parents may smile joyfully but not quite as often as those ads would have us believe. Dream babies, immaculate houses, elegant hairstyles and gowns, and reassuring, rhythmic schedules exist only in dreams—and advertisements.

The "fourth" trimester is the first three months of the baby's life. Pregnancy is normally divided into three periods, called trimesters. These trimesters culminate in the birth of the baby, the end of pregnancy; but birth is not an end, it is a beginning. The "fourth" trimester is as crucial to the baby's development and well-being as the time she spends growing within the mother's uterus. It is also a time of change—often bordering on confusion and chaos—for the parents, who must adjust to their new roles and the logistics of caring for the baby's needs. New parents, however much they love their baby, may be overwhelmed at times. The cesarean mother, whose energy reserves have been depleted, may discover that the fourth trimester is very demanding. It comes as a shock to parents to discover that their much-adored, beautiful infant has the lungs of Godzilla, the mouth of a hungry lumberjack, and the ability to go through more diapers in two days than they ordered for a whole week.

The first few months are the hardest for the parents. Both may be handicapped by lack of sleep, lack of time to be alone, and additional energy drains. Every action centers on the baby. It may seem that there are simply not enough hours in the day to care for the baby and fulfill the parents' needs as people. The mother, with her numerous roles of wife, lover, career person, and/or parent to other children, bears the brunt of the difficulties the first few months.

It is imperative that the cesarean mother have help at home for the first week or two. After the first two to six weeks, depending entirely upon the individual woman, the differences between the cesarean mother and the mother who has delivered vaginally are not so great. It's important to remember that the cesarean mother is mending her body from both childbirth and surgery. Regular household chores should be taken over by other family members, relatives, friends, or hired help. Fathers often plan to take time off when the baby is born so they can be at home that first week or two. Some fathers are able to obtain paternity leaves of absence to fulfill their essential parenting role. Grandparents, aunts, sisters, and friends usually volunteer to lend assistance. Ideally, the helper should be someone who is acceptable to both mother and father and whose help is welcomed. Some relatives, however well-intentioned, may create more problems than they solve. It's a sticky situation for the new parent who wishes to say no but who does not want to hurt a relative's feelings. If there is no graceful way to refuse an eager but unwelcome grandparent or relative, the new parents may ask the person to come for a specific period. Knowing the person will leave on a certain day is comforting. In the meantime, your relative will probably try to be as helpful as possible. More often than not, Grandmother's help is very much appreciated and the new family realizes they could not have managed without her.

Above all, when friends ask, "What can I do?" ask them to prepare a meal that just needs to be heated and served. Friends would not offer if they didn't want to help. Making dinner for the new family will allow friends to feel helpful and will save your already overburdened energies.

If possible, prepare and freeze foods while you are pregnant for use after the baby is born. Leftovers make good TV dinners with dribs of this and that. If you can afford it, you may wish to send out for food. Even a pizza or sub makes a well-rounded meal when a salad is included. When you're feeling up to it, a restaurant dinner will make a welcome change of pace. *All* parents should be encouraged to go out to a favorite restaurant sometime before the baby is three or four weeks old. It will do wonders for the mother's morale. Many men like to cook, and the father should be encouraged to help with meal preparations. For the first few weeks, use paper plates and plastic utensils. Their use is not ecologically sound, economical, or elegant, but it is helpful.

Bathing the baby can be done by the father and will provide him with a special sense of closeness to the baby. Fathers of breast-fed babies welcome this opportunity to do something essential and comforting which the mother could do but which he enjoys doing. He may take special pleasure and pride in performing this task for the baby.

The new cesarean mother should not feel guilty if she wants

to become a hermit for a few weeks. The telephone can be taken off the hook, and a No Visitors, Please sign posted on the door. One father placed such a sign on his door along with a list of chores that needed doing. Anyone who wanted to visit also helped with household tasks. As a new mother, you will need all your energy to cope with caring for yourself and the baby. When visitors do call, you may find it advantageous to remain in your gown and robe to remind visitors (and yourself!) that you should not become overtired. Loving and loved family or friends who stay too long and who do not respond to gentle hints can be told, "I'm sorry, you'll have to leave now. The doctor said Sally needs a lot of rest. It's time for her to take a nap. Won't you please come back in a few weeks?" Frequent rest breaks are advised. A rocking chair is soothing for both you and the baby—and is a good exercise that does not require a lot of energy.

Restrictions on activities for the first six weeks after delivery depend primarily on the doctor's policies and any special medical circumstances that may arise. Some doctors discharge their patients from the hospital with no limitations. These mothers leave the hospital knowing they may drive a car, go skiing, or make love if they want to. The doctor who places no restrictions is banking on the mother's body and common sense to dictate her activities. The only drawback is that some women assume because their obstetricians told them they could do anything, that they will want to do everything. They won't. Top athletes may be able to go skiing within a week after delivery, but not many cesarean mothers will have the energy even to climb two flights of stairs. The best thing to do is to take it easy and use common sense. Unfortunately, common sense is not always easy to find. Pushing yourself too hard, even if you have no restrictions, will make a longer recuperative period necessary. Do what you can—but don't overdo. And you should not feel guilty about being a little weak or becoming easily fatigued.

Just as there are doctors who place no limitations on activities, the extreme conservative approach makes everything other than going to the bathroom and feeding the baby taboo. Common prohibitions may include any or all of the following:

No Driving. This limitation may be imposed for as little as one week after discharge from the hospital, or for as long as the entire six weeks until the first checkup. The reasons are that the mother may still be weak and subject to dizzy spells. Driving also makes it easy for her to push herself to accomplish tasks for which she is not truly prepared, such as spending an hour at the supermarket or in a clothing store. There is also the risk of a seat belt irritating the fresh incision and an impaired ability to respond to a sudden emergency.

Limited Stair Climbing. If you live in a house where the only bathroom is on the second floor, to avoid climbing stairs you may wish to build a "nest" for yourself and the baby on the floor where the bathroom is located. Use a thermos or ice chest nearby to keep snacks for yourself and older children. It is much easier to keep a box of crackers stashed away in a bedroom than to have to go down to the kitchen each time your toddler or you want a snack. Carrot sticks, celery, cheese, raisins, and nuts are some other foods that are nutritious and can be prepared in advance and brought upstairs.

Not Lifting or Carrying Heavy Objects. Heavy objects include laundry, groceries, furniture and toddlers. The reason for limiting lifting or carrying is that some doctors want their postpartum cesarean mothers to avoid exertion. Your incision should be completely healed within six weeks after delivery. During those six weeks the father or a helper can do most of the lifting.

But what does a mother do when she is alone with an older child who needs help getting into her crib or down from the high chair? During your pregnancy, start teaching the older child how to climb into and out of the crib alone with the sides down, or transfer the child to a low, safe bed. If your child is agile enough, teach her to climb up and down from a booster seat placed on a regular kitchen chair. Try to plan for the times when you'll be alone with your toddler so that you can avoid lifting and carrying heavy objects as much as possible.

No Spicy Foods. This restriction is placed primarily on mothers who must stay in bed most of the time because of other problems probably unrelated to the delivery. The purpose here is to reduce the possibility of discomfort from gas. This limitation is also sometimes placed on nursing mothers. While limiting one's food is fine for upset stomachs, breast-feeding does not necessarily mean that the nursing mother will have to deprive herself of spices, garlic, onions, or chocolate. Think of the millions of women in Africa, Asia, and South America who eat such food as hot curries or chiles almost exclusively. Their babies do not seem to suffer. Experiment. If you and baby do not have problems with foods, then it is permissible to eat them.

No Tub Baths. Showers are usually permitted within a few days after delivery. For houses in which showers are not available, one compromise is to fill the tub partially with water, and then get in and wash quickly. The mother may wish to sit on a safe, low stool or even an overturned plastic pan. The important thing is to avoid contamination of the vagina by the anal area while lochia (vaginal discharge) is still being produced.

The new cesarean mother should take a bath only when someone is in the house who can help out if she needs it. Dizziness, faintness, and hot flashes may continue for some weeks after the baby's birth. Especially at first, the mother may be stiff and welcome a helping hand into and out of the tub or shower. Any new mother may find it difficult to set aside time for grooming, and the cesarean mother, who is less agile, may have difficulty bending over the sink or may become dizzy while standing in the shower to shampoo her hair.

Once the lochia has ceased, the baby may be taken into the

bath with the mother. Fathers can take the baby into the bath after the umbilical cord has healed and dropped off, which usually occurs within the first week or two of the baby's life.

No Sex for Six Weeks. Many doctors and midwives are relaxing this prohibition, but the intention is to reduce the possibility of infection. Some authorities believe the taboo comes more from Judeo-Christian tradition than from established medical fact. Many things other than penetration of the vagina by the penis constitute lovemaking and can be equally satisfying. If you cannot wait to have intercourse, two things should be kept in mind. (1) You are not alone. There are many other couples who cannot wait for the go-ahead from the doctor at the six-week checkup. A red flag will not go up during the examination to signal your transgression to the doctor, but most women confess to this "sin," even if somewhat sheepishly. (2) Even though you may not have had a period, you may still ovulate. Birth control should be used. If you are breast-feeding, a diaphragm or condom is best. Breast-feeding mothers cannot take the Pill when nursing. The diaphragm, if used, must be well lubricated with spermicidal jelly, because it may not fit properly. Be prepared! (See the section on "Sex and the Cesarean Couple" later in this chapter.)

Both mothers and babies are scheduled for checkups soon after delivery. Usually few complications occur between the hospital discharge and the postpartum visit. If there are any problems or questions, call the obstetrician.

Although six weeks is a reasonable time for the first checkup, there is a growing and positive trend for babies to have their first visit with the pediatrician within two to four weeks after birth. Although new parents should feel free to call the pediatrician at any time, many parents have not yet established a rapport with the baby's doctor and feel hesitant about telephoning for fear of appearing foolish and nervous for being concerned about a rash, a change in bowel movements, or recurrent spitting up. There is a certain reassurance that comes with visiting the pediatrician. Even if the couple are old pros at parenting, all new parents worry and fret over every diaper rash, flaky scalp, and change in the baby's eating and sleeping habits. Seeing the pediatrician at two or three weeks will set many of the parents' fears to rest before they become blown out of proportion and will stem any potentially serious problems before they become full-fledged.

Parents and babies who deliver at hospitals where policies are restrictive and unsupportive, and where Family-Centered Maternity Care is unknown, will want to implement their own family-centered touching and bonding program when they get home. Going home may be the first time the father has been able to see his baby without having to stare through a plate glass window. It may be the first time he has been able to hold her. The new mother, who has been able to have her baby only for short periods at four-hour intervals, may have little inkling of her baby's personality, feeding patterns, and sleeping habits. Breast-feeding may have been difficult to manage under such circumstances, especially in hospitals where babies are fed supplements regardless of the parents' wishes. Instead of going home with confidence and knowing what the baby is like, these parents are suddenly thrust into parenthood without preparation. The baby may be fretful at home even though she never seemed to cry while in the hospital. If medical problems have been ruled out as the cause of the baby's problem, the child may need extra love and touching. By all means, bring the baby into bed with you.

Does this mean that *all* babies who are held and touched will automatically stop crying and go to sleep? No. A fretful baby who will not sleep in a way the parents think is "proper" is the source of a great deal of worry to them. Crying may simply be the baby's way of making her presence known. Cesarean babies, who more often than not have been separated from their mothers for varying time periods, need *extra* body contact the first few days and weeks. The parents who take a baby home from the hospital where little contact has been allowed will want to give their babies additional touching, stroking, nuzzling, kissing, and cuddling. Although it is sometimes considered unfashionable by modern standards, once home from the hospital, the best place for the mother and baby the first week is in bed *together*. The more frequently the baby is offered the warmth and closeness of the mother's body (and to a lesser degree, the father's body), the more secure the baby will feel.

A happy, secure, contented baby will not cry often. Despite our hang-ups, the fact is that holding and cuddling a baby will *not* spoil her. The baby needs attention. Crying is the only way she has to get it. It may take a few weeks for the parents to determine what the baby is "saying." Sometimes it means "feed me," other times the cry means, "I'm wet and want to be changed" (although it does seem odd that a baby who has spent nine months in a wet world would mind being damp, provided she is *warm*), and sometimes it just means, "I need attention. Please love me." A baby carrier fashioned of any soft, comfortable material, or purchased (a Snugli is one excellent baby carrier), will make the baby feel secure and will leave the mother's hands free to do whatever she wants.

No matter what the parents do, there will be times when the baby's crying turns the parents' rose-colored glasses red with rage. Acceptance of the fact that the infant is almost sure to cause chaos at home for a few months will help the parents deal with the situation more realistically. There will be times when the parents are able to enjoy a nice, quiet evening together while the baby slumbers peacefully. At first, however, these times of tranquility may be few and far between. They are outnumbered by the daily hassles of dirty diapers, a hungry baby, and the usual, never-ending household chores. Maintaining a semblance of dignity and calm is often difficult for new parents.

There are benefits and joys to parenting. Most of the burden rests on the mother, and she is the one most apt to receive the benefits, but unfortunately they are not as numerous or apparent initially as the negative aspects. The circles under your eyes will disappear. You will be able to get a long, uninterrupted night's sleep . . . sometime—and, with luck, soon. There will come a time when you can take off for an outing without enough equipment and strategy planning for an African safari. And eventually you will be able to make love spontaneously without being interrupted by the baby's cries. At first, however, the baby takes precedence. To add to these frustrations, if you think that a really good mother or father *never* temporarily resents the baby's intrusion, your frustration may be compounded by guilt. Even the world's best mothers and fathers sometimes experience any or all of the feelings of frustration, anger, or resentment that a new baby may create.

To help you smooth over the fourth trimester, there are a number of good books available. The best rule of thumb when reading books on child care is to use them as a guide. The best points of each must be assimilated into your family's lifestyle and the personality of your baby.

Each baby and each parent are different. Change, chaos, disorder, and confusion are all normal conditions those first few months. Learn to flow with the river—don't try to push it. Let the dust accumulate and take the time to enjoy your baby. Cultivate the services of a good, reliable sitter, and treat yourself to an afternoon off. When you come back, you'll probably feel rejuvenated.

The father who shares in the responsibilities of caring for the children and house will gain a special closeness to his children. Both father and baby have the need and right to be with each other. A warm, loving relationship will flourish. Some fathers offer to take over all the responsibilities for an evening or afternoon, thus allowing the mother time to herself. She needs this time and will appreciate the father's caring. It may help to promote a new awareness of their relationship with each other. Today's fathers are spending more time with infant care. They are aware of the fact that tenderness does not mean a lack of manliness but rather is a reflection of their "humanness." (And mothers, if your husband does take over the cooking, cleaning, baby care, or laundry, let him do it *his* way. It may be different from your way but that doesn't matter.)

Be sure to take time out for yourself as a "person" and yourselves as a "couple." Do things you enjoy doing together. If someone offers to take the baby for a few hours or help out with the house, don't refuse this offer. Don't overlook your responsibilities to yourselves. Leave the baby with Grandma or a friend and do something special, just the two of you. If you don't have a close friend or relative to take the baby for a few hours, it may be possible to arrange a swap with a friend. You spend a certain number of hours with her baby in exchange for a few of her hours with yours.

At one time or another, most parents say, "I could just throw the kid out the window, I'm so mad." But if that is the only way they feel, or if they say they want to do away with the child and really mean it, professional help is imperative. If the aggravations of parenthood are overwhelming or persistent, professional counseling is essential.

Many communities now offer groups for the education and support of new parents. They may be postpartum groups that have developed as an outgrowth of a prepared childbirth program, or they may have formed as the result of parental interest. Some of these groups have regular meetings as well as supplemental hot lines or listening-ear services. When a parent feels ready to blow up, a phone number can be dialed and negative feelings, questions or concerns vented at the person at the other end of the line—instead of at the baby. If there is no such program in your area, a friend may be able to help.

For first-time parents, this chapter may seem unnecessarily gloomy. Veteran parents will be aware of the realities and responsibilities of caring for a newborn. Parenthood is an

Baby Equipment and Clothing

That old Yankee saying, "Use it up, wear it out, make it do, or do without" seems all but lost in our disposable, throwaway, plastic society. Everything from automobiles to diapers is designed with obsolescence in mind.

It isn't necessary to spend hundreds (sometimes thousands) of dollars on the newest, biggest, best, shiniest baby equipment and clothing. You can outfit your baby and provide for all her furniture needs without spending a fortune.

Baby equipment and furniture can be swapped or borrowed. Classified ads in local newspapers and bargain weeklies are good sources. Yard, barn, and garage sales are excellent places to purchase used baby items for a mere fraction of their original cost.

Baby clothes can also be found in yard sales, flea markets, and thrift shops. Check the clothing over carefully because sometimes it is stained and ripped. If you don't mind, your baby won't. A complete, attractive layette can usually be purchased. When cleaned it will look as though it came from the town's most expensive store.

The two most important items your baby will need are a firm mattress and a safe car carrier. The car seat should be sturdy and face toward the back of the car when installed. A worn, too-soft mattress is bad for the infant's soft, rapidly growing bones. A piece of foam two or three inches thick makes an excellent, inexpensive mattress, can be cut to any size or shape, and is ideal if you've just bought a delightful but eccentrically shaped antique crib or cradle.

Strollers, musical swings, cribs, cradles, mobiles, back carriers, and all other items are usually readily available— although some items are more in demand than others (a used Snugli is hard to find), so you may have to shop around a bit. You'll be saving money and recycling at the same time!

awesome responsibility. Real babies are wonderful and precious. They also wet, cry, get hungry, sleep (but not always at
the most convenient hours), and fret. There is pleasure and joy
that comes from holding the baby in your arms. There is pride
and happiness when the baby smiles at you for the first time.
There is something very special and fulfilling about seeing part
of you reflected in your baby's features and habits. Once you've
made it through the first three or four months, you will
probably forget—or at least gloss over—the trials and tribula-
tions of this fourth trimester.

SEX AND THE CESAREAN COUPLE

As a new mother, you may find that your interest in
sex is at an all-time low. Childbirth via surgery, the demands of
the newborn, the lack of a full night's sleep without interrup-
tion for at least one feeding, and caring for the house and older
children as well as the new baby may be so draining that you
have neither the time nor the inclination to make love, at least
for a while. The baby's father may not be the type to pressure
you about sex, but you may pressure yourself into wanting to
please your partner, even though you're not feeling up to it.

Some couples do make love either with or without the
doctor's permission before the six weeks are up. The woman's
vagina may not lubricate as well as it did before she had the
baby. Lack of lubrication is a normal course of events brought
about by the hormonal changes of giving birth, but it may cause
discomfort or pain. K-Y Jelly or any other brand of lubricant
rubbed on the penis or vagina, or both, before intercourse will
overcome the lack of lubrication and make penetration easier.

During pregnancy it is a good idea to explore how you will
deal with contraception afterward. Birth control is necessary if
you wish to space your pregnancies and are not ready for
permanent sterilization. Finding a suitable temporary method
is difficult. Prior to the six-week checkup, the mother who

wants to use an IUD will not have had one inserted. A diaphragm that fit properly before pregnancy may not offer the same amount of protection now, for the opening in the cervix can stretch somewhat during pregnancy even in cesarean mothers. If you do use your old diaphragm, be sure to apply lots of spermicidal jelly. Condoms are acceptable methods of birth control, although some people find them distasteful and/or do not like them because they may reduce sensation. Withdrawal before ejaculation is not satisfactory, because sperm may be present in pre-ejaculatory fluid. Foams and spermicidal jelly used singly are anything but fail-safe. Birth control pills, of course, cannot be taken by nursing mothers because the hormones they contain will be transmitted to the baby. Plan ahead!

The mother's scar can be a source of concern. Won't it be ruptured during lovemaking? Does it make the woman less appealing to her mate? The classical cesarean skin incision from bellybutton to pubis is particularly blatant. If the woman's pubic hair has been shaved, she may feel like a plucked chicken, which further lowers her morale. As the pubic hair grows back, it itches or prickles, a sensation that may be irritating as she rubs her body against her mate's. The newly delivered cesarean mother feels particularly vulnerable at this time, when her incision is fresh and her pubic hair shorn. Rupture of the scar is all but impossible, but its presence is a reminder to both the mother and father that this is a time to be gentle and considerate.

Women's concerns about the scar are sometimes valid. A very few are initially repulsed by it. Most men are understanding and accept it with even greater ease than the mother herself. The best thing for the couple to do is talk about their feelings openly and honestly soon after the baby is born. The "problem" may not be a problem at all, except in the mother's mind. She needs reassurance that she is no less lovely and appealing than before.

Making love can be relaxing and fulfilling—at a time when

the mother and father are able to share the closeness and warmth that can only be expressed sexually—or it can be a time of resentment and frustration for both partners. If the mother feels pressured into making love before she is ready, if the baby starts to fuss right in the middle of things, the mother is apt to be so distracted that her mind wanders.

The baby's father needs to exhibit patience, understanding, and tact—but he may find these concerns for the mother's welfare difficult to express if he has been unable to fulfill his desire for weeks or even months. Few doctors, except in special cases, routinely prohibit sex during the last six weeks of pregnancy, but there are exceptions.

During pregnancy the mother may have felt more amorous than usual. After the baby is born her desire to make love may be lessened. This temporary decrease is partially due to physical fatigue from the stress of surgery, childbirth, and the extra demands the new baby places on her time and energy. It is normal, it is natural, but it can be disturbing to both parents. The father may secretly resent the baby for intruding and requiring so much attention. The mother may have these feelings, too.

Finding the time to make love may require more planning and cooperation than it did before. And the parents may wish to express their love in other forms of pleasuring rather than intercourse. Getting back to "normal" may take time, but it can be achieved. Understanding on the part of both parents will make this transition easier.

POSTPARTUM EXERCISES

The cesarean mother is apt to believe that her stomach muscles have been severed and that she can never hope to have a flat stomach again. This myth is widespread, inaccurate, and convenient—why exercise when it won't help anyway?

Right after delivery, the new mother may feel like Twiggy.

However, when she gets on the scales at home, or tries to put on a comfortable pair of slacks, she may realize that she isn't quite as thin as she thought she was. It takes at least a few months for her to lose every ounce of weight gained during pregnancy, and even if she does get back to prepregnancy size, there may still be some extra, very discouraging flab in the way.

You should discuss with your doctor any diet planned for weight loss and any exercise program designed for reducing flab and extra inches. Generally, once the mother has had her six-week checkup, it is safe to begin an exercise program. In the meantime, the mother can use a rocking chair to promote circulation and, after a week or so when she is less bothered by the incision, she can "walk" by pressing her feet against a pillow at the end of her bed while pulling her stomach in and out. This exercise also promotes circulation and will help the muscles of the abdomen tone up. The abdominal tightening exercise will help, too.

After your obstetrician has given the go-ahead, almost any exercise program is acceptable. Elizabeth Noble's *Essential Exercises for the Childbearing Year* offers excellent post-cesarean exercises. Some organizations offer classes of swimming, slimnastics, and postpartum exercises. Walking, bike riding, tennis, and jogging (with the doctor's all-clear signal) also promote muscle tone. Doing sit-ups, deep knee bends, and running-in-place will also help. Just be certain to check with your doctor and don't overdo any exercises.

HUMAN BONDING:
THE IMPORTANCE OF TOUCHING
AND THE ADVANTAGES
OF BREAST-FEEDING

Caesarean-delivered babies suffer from a number of disadvantages from the moment they are delivered. . . .

It may be conjectured that the disadvantages, among other things, from which caesarean-delivered babies suffer, compared with vaginally delivered babies, are to a significant extent related to the failure of adequate cutaneous stimulation which they have undergone. . . .

The moment it is born, the cord is cut or clamped, the child is exhibited to its mother, and then it is taken away. . . .

The two people who need each other at this time, more than they will at any other in their lives, are separated from one another, prevented from continuing the development of a symbiotic relationship which is so crucially necessary for the further development of both of them.

During the whole of pregnancy the mother has been elaborately prepared, in every possible way, for the continuation of the symbiotic union between herself and her child, to minister to its dependent needs in the manner for which she alone is best prepared. It is not simply that the baby needs her, but that both need each other. The mother needs the baby quite as much as the baby needs its mother. The biological unity maintained by the mother and conceptus throughout pregnancy does not cease at birth but becomes—indeed, is naturally designed to become—even more intensified and interoperative than during uterogestation. Giving birth to her child, the mother's interest and involvement in its welfare is deepened and reinforced. Her whole organism has been readied to minister to its needs, to caress it, to make loving sounds to it, to nurse it at the breast. . . .

During the birth process mother and infant have had a somewhat trying time. At birth each clearly requires the reassurance of the other's presence. The reassurance for the mother lies in the sight of her baby, its first cry, and in its closeness to her body. For the baby it consists in the contact with and warmth of the mother's body, the support in her cradled arms, the caressing it receives, and the suckling at her breast, the welcome to the "bosom of the family." These are words, but they refer to very real psycho-physiological conditions.[1]

Modern science is just now recognizing what so-called primitive cultures have known and practiced for centuries: that the newborn human infant needs to be stroked and touched as much as she needs to be nourished and kept warm. If she is to develop into a happy, secure, intelligent person, it is important to keep the parents (especially the mother) and baby together as much as possible from the moment of birth and to offer the opportunity for them to have early, frequent, close physical contact. These are not "niceties." They are essential.

"Human bonding" is the term used by professionals for the very complex processes that establish deep and lasting emotional ties between parents and their offspring. Many assume that parental love comes in an immediate, intense, blinding, automatic, almost magical flash. It doesn't. The first few days and weeks of the infant's life, extending for the next six to nine months, are a crucial period when the roots of love are planted.

From these roots, the child will flourish or fail to thrive. Human bonding is a period of adjustment, a sort of ritual recognition, a "welcome to the world" ceremony with both immediate and long-range consequences. Early, frequent contact between the parents and baby will lay the foundation for the nurturing and care of the baby's physical and emotional needs. Bonding is a term that encompasses acceptance of the baby by the parents (and vice versa), the way the parents and baby relate to each other, and the *quality* of the care extended to the baby. The baby who is loved, stroked, admired, gazed at, talked to, held close, and cuddled is the child who will thrive and who will grow into a secure, well-adjusted adult human being.

Babies pick up messages from parents. These messages may be verbal (oohing and aahing, cooing, or singing a lullaby are positive messages; a harsh, loud voice is a negative one) or tactile (the infant can sense from the way she is handled whether the message is positive or negative). The baby who is born into a warm, demonstrative atmosphere with a significant person, usually the mother, lavishing affection on her will have a firm foundation on which to build future human relationships. Many factors determine the quality of the initial contact between the mother and baby. This initial contact is of great importance. Yet for the cesarean family, outside influences may greatly hinder or impede the establishment of parental-infant bonding. For example, an emergency cesarean, performed after a long and difficult labor, will have depleted the mother's energy reserves. Her physical and emotional condition (for example, if she is in great pain, frightened, or confused by the events around her) will inhibit the maternal-infant bonding process. This reaction is understandable, and the mother is justified in being somewhat more egocentric than she would have been had the labor and delivery taken place easily. If the delivery has taken place with general anesthesia, it will be many hours before the mother and baby are united. Even if spinal or epidural anesthetic has been used, the mother whose baby is whisked away with only a fleeting glimpse (or none at all) will not be able to initiate the maternal-infant bonding and attachment processes immediately as is ideal. When parents and babies are separated for many hours or days, the bonding process is delayed. Hospitals with rigid four-hour feeding schedules and limited Family-Centered Maternity Care (if it is provided at all) hinder the bonding and touching rituals.

It is usually easier to initiate the bonding and touching processes in a vaginal delivery. To illustrate, here is a description of an "ideal" vaginal delivery (and few vaginal deliveries are as easy and straightforward as the one presented here).

The "ideal" vaginal delivery takes place after a 12-hour labor in which the mother has had no medication. She has been comfortable and in control of the situation by using one of the breathing methods (such as Bing, Lamaze, or Kitzinger) learned in prenatal classes. Her husband has been with her in the birthing room throughout labor as coach and supporter. Within seconds of the birth, the infant is placed in the mother's arms by the happy father. The mother immediately breast-feeds the baby, the father beams and takes pictures. The parents and their baby are the center of attention. The happy family leaves the Alternative Birth Center within less than a day after delivery.

The baby is not relegated to a separate room but is kept in the parents' room. At night, the parents have no hesitation about bringing the baby into bed with them, knowing that parents have an "automatic alarm system" that prevents them from rolling over on the baby. When the baby awakens at night for feedings, the father changes her diapers and the mother turns on her side with pillows propped around her to feed the baby. No chilly trips to the kitchen, no waiting for a bottle to heat. The baby usually falls asleep in the mother's arms, and she can simply lay the child down beside her before she falls asleep.

During the day, the baby is frequently carried about in a

Snugli. The mother's hands are free and she can move about comfortably. Meanwhile, the baby is reassured by the closeness of the mother's body, the sound of her familiar heartbeat and voice. The family takes hikes or bike trips with the baby safely strapped in. The father spends several hours a day with the baby, playing, changing diapers, talking with her, bathing her, enjoying their child.

How does this illustration of an ideal vaginal delivery and postpartum period compare with the average cesarean experience? The parents may not have been together the entire time but may have had a number of separations from each other, even with Family-Centered Maternity Care. For varying periods of time, it is still frequently necessary for the baby to be cared for not at the parents' side but in a special care nursery. Certainly, the newly delivered cesarean mother is unable to move easily and comfortably for the first week or so after delivery. Because she cannot go home from the hospital twelve hours after surgery, her hospital stay is longer and she requires more help and care from the hospital staff and her support person. Breast-feeding may be difficult to initiate, especially since cesarean mothers are less mobile and take postoperative pain medication more frequently. There's greater difficulty getting into bed, holding the baby, changing sides while nursing, burping, and diapering. At home, carrying the baby during the first few weeks is made difficult by the incision, fatigue, and postoperative stress.

What can parents and hospital personnel do to improve the situation for cesarean families? How can early, frequent bonding and touching be established for these parents and babies? Some suggestions for more positive approaches and more supportive care, which have already been instituted in a growing number of hospitals, are:

     1. Ideally, unless there are medical contraindications, the mother should be awake for the baby's birth. Being awake will enable her to establish immediate contact with the

infant. Seeing one's baby is a right, not a privilege. The baby is not "hospital property."

2. If the umbilical cord is long enough, the obstetrician could hold the baby up over the screen so the mother can see her seconds-old newborn all wet and covered with vernix. Parents have envisioned this moment for many years, and their desire to see it has been reinforced by books, films, and articles. It is a precious sight and one to which cesarean parents are entitled.

3. Cesarean parents should always be allowed to be together for the delivery itself, regardless of the type of anesthesia used. If the mother has spinal or epidural anesthesia, this is a wonderful time of sharing. If general anesthesia is unavoidable because of contraindications, then by all means the father or significant other should be present to take pictures, if desired, and to be able to relate the story of their baby's birth to the mother afterward.

4. In addition to the father and/or another person chosen by the mother, it is now suggested that "labor attendants" (LA's) be present as well. These assistants are there to provide support, encouragement, and aid to *both* parents during birth. For cesareans, it is suggested that labor attendants also be permitted into the delivery room.

5. Before the baby is placed in the warmer unit, a nurse or pediatrician should give the parents at least an up-close glimpse of their baby. It is important to resuscitate the baby, clean mucus from the mouth, give additional oxygen, take the Apgar ratings, and keep the baby from becoming chilled; but a quick viewing can and should take place first.

6. The baby care unit should always be placed within eyesight of the mother. After months of waiting for this day, seeing the back of a doctor's or nurse's head and being told your baby is fine simply will not do. Only the sight of her child will reassure the mother.

7. As soon as the baby has been immediately cared

for, she should be presented to the father and mother for physical contact. Even if the mother's hands are not free, she can still touch the baby with her face and caress it with her eyes. This kissing, nuzzling, touching, stroking, and smelling will help release the mother's maternal responses and will reassure her.

8. The father, when present, can cuddle the baby close and talk with the mother. If the father is not or does not wish to be present, and the mother does not have a significant other with her for the birth, the nurse or pediatrician can help mother and baby initiate bonding.

9. Erythromycin or silver nitrate is routinely administered to the eyes of all newborns. You have the right to refuse the use of these drops if it's not a law in your state. If you do give consent, by all means request that administration of the drops be put off as long as possible so that the mother and baby have time to establish eye contact. Erythromycin is much less irritating than silver nitrate but, even so, both make it difficult for your baby to look at you.

10. For parents who wish to have a Leboyer-style birth, it is possible to achieve the spirit of this method during a cesarean delivery. The Leboyer method is named in honor of Dr. Frederic Leboyer, the French physician who promoted the benefits of welcoming new babies into the world in a very gentle manner. His method advocates dim lighting, soft, soothing voices, massage of the newborn in a bath of warm water or on the mother's abdomen immediately after birth, and an over-all calm and peaceful reception. With a cesarean delivery, the lights cannot be dimmed in an operating room and the mother may be unable to hold her brand new infant until she returns to the recovery room. But the father or a support person can give the baby a gentle massage within eyesight of the mother after she has had a chance to touch and kiss her baby.

11. Reuniting babies with their parents (and possi-

bly siblings and grandparents) in the recovery room as soon as possible will also release many of the maternal responses and will reassure the family. For the infant, being held in the mother's arms will replicate the warmth and reassurance of the intrauterine environment and will promote closeness and security.

12. The condition of cesarean babies should be judged on an individual basis. Until recently, all cesarean babies were placed in the special care nursery for observation regardless of their birth weight, Apgar score, temperature, or overall condition. This tradition sprang from the high incidence of respiratory distress among cesarean-delivered babies. Now, thanks to prenatal tests to determine fetal maturity and well-being, and improved medical, surgical, and neonatal techniques and equipment, the cesarean baby has a greater-than-ever opportunity to be born healthy and full term—especially when a trial of labor has taken place.

Parents should consult with a pediatrician before delivery to determine what policies their hospitals and doctors have. Engaging the services of a sympathetic pediatrician in advance of delivery may enable you to hold your healthy, unendangered baby soon after delivery rather than hours or days later. While no one would advocate anything but the best care for an endangered infant, it is now possible to have a perfectly healthy cesarean baby who does not need the special care nursery.

13. Giving the mother an opportunity to begin breast-feeding soon after birth will give the baby the benefit of skin contact and colostrum.

14. During the family's reunion in the recovery room, the staff will want to maintain a low profile and to intrude only if the parents ask for assistance or advice.

15. When central nurseries, separate from the maternity floor or recovery room, are used, the mother needs constant assurances from the staff and the baby's father that her child is alive and well. This reassurance is just as important

for mothers who have been reunited with their infants in the recovery room as it is for those who cannot hold their babies for many hours. An instantly developed picture of the child will reassure her further.

16. Once the mother has begun rooming-in (and later at home) she may wish to keep the room fairly dim for the baby who has lived for nine months in a warm, dark world. Rocking chairs, unfortunately not found in most American hospitals, are soothing and relaxing for mother and baby.

17. Fathers should be encouraged, through flexible, accommodating hospital policies, to take part in caring for and nurturing their infants. Support from the hospital staff with a "it's so nice you're here" attitude (as opposed to "fathers are always in the way") will promote the father's attachment to the child.

If the cesarean family is unable to establish immediate eye and skin contact, or cannot care for the child as they would like to in the hospital because of medical reasons or hospital practice, they should reassure themselves that they will be able to make up for lost time and nurture the child according to their own wishes once they are home. A parent who is highly motivated will overcome any obstacle.

And the baby who is loved and cherished, touched and kissed, will thrive. It has been said that the price we human beings pay for our higher intellect is a loss of instinct. This seems to be particularly true with regard to current birthing practices and child care attitudes. But the tide is turning. Parents are beginning to trust themselves and their instincts more. Your baby knows what she wants and needs. And you know how to provide it. Some things have to be learned—such as how to fasten a diaper securely on a wiggling baby—but most things will come automatically. If our babies could talk, they might say, "See me, feel me, touch me, love me," and that's just what many parents are doing. They're looking at their babies, talking to them, carrying them about in infant carriers, holding them close in their arms, bringing them into bed with them, breast-feeding them, and doing all the things babies need and want. As parents, we want to give our babies the best possible start in life. A healthy human being is not just one who cries at birth and who "pinks up" rapidly, but one who as an adult is physically, neurologically, and emotionally sound. And the ways to achieve that well-being begin at birth. Not everything can be measured in quantitative scientific terms. In human terms, touching and bonding will improve the quantity and quality of the life of the human child.

> It is through body contact with the mother that the child makes its first contact with the world, through which he is enfolded in a new dimension of experience, the experience of the world of the other. It is this . . . that provides the essential source of comfort, security, warmth, and increasing aptitude for the new experiences. . . .
>
> What the child requires if it is to prosper . . . is to be handled and carried, caressed and cuddled, and cooed to, even if it isn't breastfed. It is handling, the carrying, the caressing and that cuddling that we would here emphasize, for it would seem that even in the absence of a great deal else, these are the reassuringly basic experiences that the infant must enjoy if it is to survive in some semblance of health. Extreme sensory deprivation in other respects, such as light and sound, can be survived, as long as the sensory experiences of the skin are maintained.
>
> To be tender, loving and caring, human beings must be tenderly loved and cared for in their earliest years, from the moment they are born. Held in the arms of their mothers, caressed, cuddled, and comforted, the familiar human environment . . . is found. . . .[2]

WHY BREAST-FEEDING IS OF SPECIAL
SIGNIFICANCE TO CESAREAN MOTHERS
AND BABIES

Breast-feeding is not only *possible* after a cesarean delivery; in my view, it is *preferable* for cesarean mothers and babies.

Rarely are cesarean mothers too weak or infants too ill to be breast-fed. The "problems" associated with breast-feeding come primarily from societal attitudes that there is something "dirty" or "old-fashioned" about it. Hospitals are not immune to those pressures and may have restrictive policies that restrain rather than encourage and promote breast-feeding. The new mother has many questions about feeding her baby. To overcome any hesitation she may have, she needs information, encouragement, and understanding. The mother who asks her obstetrician, nurse, or pediatrician about breast-feeding does not want to hear, "Well, you can if you want to. It's really up to you." She knows that already. She wants information. She may need only a bit of encouragement to convince her that breast-feeding is proper, best for her baby, and natural. Doctors and nurses who feel comfortable discussing breast-feeding and respond with, "Of course you want to know about it. It's best for you and baby . . ." are to be commended. Unfortunately many health care professionals are just as confused and uptight as some parents. Often the most positive, informative assistance the new or expectant mother can obtain comes from the many excellent books on the subject or from groups such as La Leche League, an organization with chapters in many cities and towns throughout the country. Any parent interested in learning more about breast-feeding is encouraged to attend a meeting of a local chapter or write to La Leche League Headquarters at 9616 Minneapolis Avenue, Franklin Park, Illinois 60131. You don't have to become a member to attend local meetings. La

Leche League is the best and often the only place where parents can turn to find out about breast-feeding.

In the United States, an estimated one-third of mothers breast-feed their babies. This low statistic is both shocking and disquieting. Why so few? Who or what is to be blamed? And what are the special advantages of breast-feeding as they apply to the cesarean mother and baby?

The cesarean baby, who may not have had the beneficial stimulation of labor, who has not passed through the birth canal, and who may have been separated from the mother immediately after birth, has special handicaps. To make up for these handicaps, cesarean babies may need the mother's milk even more than vaginally delivered babies—although breast-feeding is certainly the best way to nourish any infant.

Breast-feeding, in addition to its nutritional benefits, is a natural intimate relationship between mother and baby. If the mother feels uncomfortable with her body or its functions, she may find breast-feeding difficult, if not impossible. One slogan of our era should be, "Let's get our breasts out of the pages of girlie magazines and into our babies' mouths." It is because of this emphasis on breasts as sex symbols and objects of fantasy, rather than as sources of nourishment and comfort to our children, that some people regard breast-feeding as "smutty." Mothers who breast-feed their babies may find it absurd—if not vulgar—for a mother to shove a plastic bottle into a baby's mouth. Yet many others are conditioned to think that it is pornographic to use breasts for their natural function. How sad.

One distinct advantage to breast-feeding is that it is a built-in system of immunizing the baby against many diseases. This immunization begins with the first few drops of colostrum the baby takes the first time she nurses. In addition, "menstrual bleeding tends to be heavier and longer-lasting when the mother does not breast-feed, and, as a consequence of the heavier bleeding, the mother's energies tend to be somewhat depleted."³ Certainly, the cesarean mother who is already prone to exhaustion does not need this additional drain.

Breast-feeding is a good but *not* fail-safe method of birth control. La Leche League advises that protection from conception while breast-feeding is excellent in the first few months *if* the baby is *totally* nursed, without supplemental feedings or the use of pacifier or thumb. Total breast-feeding of this magnitude is unrealistic for many of today's women. It is not always possible, or, in some cases, preferable. A woman who breast-feeds her baby completely, to the exclusion of any supplemental feedings, pacification, or thumbsucking, may not have much time to worry about the need for contraception. She may be so preoccupied with feeding the baby that she is too fatigued or busy to care about making love, especially if she has a "barracuda" who likes to nurse frequently and for long periods. La Leche League suggests that new mothers be fitted with a diaphragm or ask their partners to use condoms in addition to the protection of breast-feeding. Birth control pills cannot be taken by nursing women, because the hormones in them may be passed on to the baby. But this is the only method that cannot be used.

It is often said that all women are born with a "natural" mothering instinct: the instant the mother looks at her baby, she supposedly will melt with love, caring, understanding, and know-how. This "natural" instinct is fallacious. While it may be true that all women had this instinct for preserving the species in early evolutional stages (before childbirth became a pathological "sickness" and child care a complicated process comprehended only by "experts"), love and acceptance of the baby may not come in a divine flash. Hours, days, or even weeks may pass before the mother feels truly maternal and confident of her capability to care for her child. The cesarean mother who has been under general anesthesia for the birth, and/or who is kept "doped up" for days afterward and separated from her baby, is more inclined to feel a sense of detachment from the bundle presented to her as "her" baby. Breast-feeding may enhance and promote the confidence she needs to care for and love her newborn.

Cesarean mothers may be prone to difficulties in relating to their babies initially. They were not able to push their babies out by themselves, and they have been separated from them for hours or days. In addition, their general physical condition the first few days may make it very difficult for them to respond to their babies. There may be initial feelings of unreality or disassociation and of disbelief ("You say that this baby is mine. How do I know that it's mine?"). Being able to breast-feed her baby—something special she can do—may enable her to finalize her pregnancy and accept her offspring.

There are important aspects of breast-feeding that are unique to cesarean mothers. For the cesarean mother who anticipated a natural vaginal delivery and sharing the event with the baby's father, there may be a sense of failure. The mother may have felt totally uninvolved in the birth, thereby delaying the mothering process, which further compounds her sense of failure or guilt. Breast-feeding is something most woman *can* accomplish. The rare exceptions are women with renal disease, cancer, tuberculosis, heart problems, and those who are on certain anticoagulant drugs. Breast-feeding carries a special, profound significance for the cesarean mother. It is something she can do successfully, and it is natural, womanly, and best for baby.

Cesarean delivery is not in itself a contraindication for breast-feeding. But the initiation of feedings may be complicated as a result of weakness, fatigue, pain, medication, and a lack of mobility. *It can be done.* If the mother wishes to breast-feed, she should do so by all means. She and the baby have nothing to lose by at least trying. They have everything to gain. It may take two or even three weeks for the mother to feel comfortable, confident, and relaxed while nursing. Discouragement comes easily. Encouragement and support are harder to come by. The cesarean mother who chooses to breast-feed, and who sticks to it, is a very special person. She will be the one out of five mothers who gives birth by cesarean, and one out of three who breast-feeds.

The decision to breast-feed is also influenced by the father. If he thinks there is something wrong with it, or if he is afraid that it will require too much of the mother's time and take attention away from him, he may try to discourage the mother. He is probably the type of man who is jealous of the baby for using a part of the mother's body over which he feels he has total control and access.

Choosing to breast-feed should not be a decision accompanied by fanfare, hoopla, and nagging fears—but sometimes it is. It is so natural and so right that it should not be the subject of debate in books (or in chapters within books) devoted to it—but it is. It should be thought of as the only right way. Instead of the encouragement they need, mothers may find their paths blocked by doctors, nurses, family, friends, and even the baby's father. Sometimes all the mother needs to overcome her hesitation is assurance that breast-feeding is best for baby and that she has the support and encouragement of people she trusts.

Babies are very different in the way they feed. Some babies are leisurely nursers and sometimes appear uninterested in feeding. Others may be real go-getters and eager beavers (the "barracuda" type) who suck the minute the nipple reaches the mouth and who want to be fed often and for long periods of time.

Nursing does place extra nutritional demands upon the mother. If you're a nursing mother, drink at least 10 glasses of liquid a day (water, beer, milk, or juices), and try to have at least 80 grams of protein a day. Liver and greens such as spinach will also add to your iron intake, a vital nutrient for nursing mothers. Many mothers suggest keeping a thermos full of ice water or juice beside the bed at night. You won't have to get out of bed when you awaken thirsty—and you will probably be thirsty for as long as you nurse your baby.

The closeness breast-feeding affords is without equal. The benefits to the baby are tremendously important. And if the mother feels that she is a failure or less womanly because she hasn't been able to push the baby out herself, she can do something that is right and natural after all. The mother who breast-feeds does not have to justify her decision. But perhaps mothers who don't even consider it should ask themselves, "Why not?"

SOLID FOODS

Another question parents frequently ask is, When should the baby be started on solid foods? Naturally, each baby is different, and the pediatrician takes this individuality into account when advising new parents on which solid foods should be started. It is generally agreed that the newborn human infant receives little or no benefit from solid food before the sixth to eighth week of life.

Until as recently as twenty or thirty years ago, babies were not placed on solid foods at such early ages. This recent innovation seems to have started following World War II as a result of pressure exerted on pediatricians by parents who thought it a status symbol to feed their babies solid foods at earlier and earlier ages. Some pediatricians and parents now place babies on solids as early as one week! The new mother, thinking she is doing the right thing, with or without the encouragement of the pediatrician, sometimes feels very proud about how soon she gives her infant solids. Such early feeding of solid foods is to be discouraged almost without exception.

The newborn's stomach lining is not adequately prepared to ingest anything other than colostrum and breast milk. Both contain elements that coat the lining of the baby's stomach and prepare the infant for other foods eventually. Many parents and professionals now believe that artificial feedings (formula), early solid foods, and rigid feeding schedules may account for more problems (such as colic, diarrhea, or constipation) than any other factor.

Until about the sixth month of life, the infant can obtain all substances needed to promote growth from the mother's milk. After the fifth month, the infant may need additional iron, either from vitamin supplements or foods. It is interesting to note that the infant usually begins to cut teeth at about the same time. Teeth may be Nature's signal that it is now time to begin solid foods.

If the baby is fussy all the time, and the parents have tried everything in their power to calm her (such as frequent holding and rocking), the pediatrician may advise supplementing the infant's intake with solid foods before the sixth month. Usually the pediatrician also advises the parents to observe the baby for a few weeks after solid foods have been started. If the infant seems to improve, that is, is less fussy, then solid foods may be the answer. However, if there is no improvement, and the infant has been thoroughly examined to rule out other medical causes for the fussiness, the parents may continue or discontinue feeding the infant solids.

It is now known that the baby who grows fat on solid food and formula is likely to become an overweight adult. Thus, breast-feeding is preferable to feeding a baby formula and solid foods.

When to start the infant on solids is a matter for the parents and the pediatrician to decide. If the doctor tells you to start feeding solids because your infant is not getting enough nourishment from your milk, it's difficult for parents to argue with such advice. The parents are apt to feel guilty and remiss in their duties if they don't start giving the infant solid foods—and perhaps just as guilty if they do. If your doctor recommends early solids (at one week or one month or whenever) and you have strong feelings about it, by all means talk to your doctor about them. There may be special reasons for the decision. As a general rule, if the baby is breast-fed at least six times within a twenty-four-period, takes vitamins to ensure an adequate supply of all nutrients (especially iron), gains weight slowly but surely, and has at least six wet diapers per day, the baby is progressing well and the parents should not be concerned.

13

HISTORY AND EVOLUTION
OF THE CESAREAN DELIVERY

> Birth in this extraordinary
> manner, as described in
> ancient mythology and
> legend, was believed to
> confer supernatural powers
> and elevate the heros so
> born above ordinary
> mortals.[1]

How is it that we have been able to arrive at a procedure that is so safe that it is preferred to a long, complicated, or difficult vaginal delivery? If it's so "good," why was it not used more often even as recently as five or ten years ago?

The cesarean as it is performed today is the product of centuries of trial and error, experimentation, and far more failures than successes. The operation is now safe and relatively pain free. With anesthesia, antisepsis, improved surgical techniques and equipment, blood transfusions (if necessary), prenatal tests to determine fetal maturity and well-being, and advances in the care of the newborn, both mother and father can approach the delivery with confidence, knowing there is minimal risk involved and great promise of a safe delivery, comfortable recovery period, and a healthy baby.

Ask anyone where the term "cesarean section" comes from. They'll tell you that Julius Caesar was the first person to be delivered in this manner, and that we have named the operation in his honor. This belief is most assuredly untrue. Surgical delivery was known for at least one thousand years

The Death of Queen Jane

Queen Jane lay in labour for six days or more,
'Till the women and midwives had given her o'er:
"O if ye be friends as women should be,
Ye would send for the surgeon and bring Henry to me!"

The surgeon was sent for, he came with great speed,
King Henry arrived, and he was aggrieved,
The king held Jane's hand as he sat by her side,
"What aileth thee Janie, what aileth my bride?"

"King Henry, King Henry, if kind Henry ye be,
You'll pay heed to the doctor and set our babe free!
King Henry, my beloved, will ye do this for me?
Let them open my side to save our sweet baby!"

"Queen Jane, dearest Janie, that I'll never do,
To so open your side would mean sure death for you!
"Dear Henry, my husband, this I do implore:
To at least save our baby, tho I'll be no more."

The doctor gave her rich caudle,* but into death slipped she,
They pierced open her side and set the babe free.
The babe it was christened and put out to nurse,
Whilst royal Queen Janie lay cold on the earth.

Six knights and six lords bore her corpse through the grounds,
Six dukes followed after in black mourning gowns.
So black was the mourning, so black were their bands,
So black were the weapons they held in their hands.

The bells they were muffled, and mournful did play,
Whilst royal Queen Janie was buried that day.
The flower of England was laid cold in the clay,
Whilst royal King Henry came weeping away.

They mourned in the kitchen, they mourned in the hall,
But royal King Henry mourned longest of all.
"Fare thee well my beloved," he grieved his heart sore,
"The Red Rose of England shall flourish no more."

*Caudle: Sweetened wine.

Adapted from Child ballad #170.

Jane Seymour, wife of Henry VIII, died shortly after giving birth to Prince Edward in October of 1537. Actually, she did not have a cesarean delivery although folk history credits her with one. She died of childbed fever two weeks after delivery.

before Caesar's lifetime—although it was seldom performed on living women. *Williams Obstetrics* offers this explanation:

> It has been generally asserted that Julius Caesar (100–44 B.C.) was brought into the world by this [surgical] means and obtained his name from the manner in which he was delivered (*a caeso matris utero*). . . . In the Roman law, as codified by Numa Pompilius (762–715 B.C.), it was ordered that the operation should be performed upon women dying in the last few weeks of pregnancy in hope of saving the child. This *lex regia,* as it was called at first, under the emperors became the *lex caessarea,* and the procedure itself became known as the *caesarean* operation. . . .[2]

> The term probably is derived from the Latin, *partus caesareus,* from *caedere,* to cut. The term caesarean section, therefore, is really a redundancy. There is no evidence to show that Julius Caesar was thus delivered. Caesones (children delivered by section from their dead mothers) were known long before Caesar's time, and the operation was not performed on the living in Rome. Caesar's mother was alive at the time of his wars, as is proved by his letters to her.[3]

One of the earliest mythological references to the cesarean delivery is the birth of Aesculapius, historically regarded as the god of medicine and the son of Apollo and Coronis.[4] Variations of the tale credit either Eileitheyria, midwife to the gods at that time (1300 B.C.), or Apollo with removing the child from the mother's uterus as her body was being carried to the funeral pyre.

As expected, the one consistency I found in researching the cesarean procedure through history has been inconsistency. For example, some texts claim that the ancient Egyptians make no recorded references to this surgical method of delivery. Others, such as *Principles and Practice of Obstetrics* (1943 edition) claim:

> Cesarean section on the dead woman has been done for ages, possibly even by the early Egyptians, and the operation is referred to in the myths and folklore of European races. . . . Cesarean section on the living is of more recent date, though it is more than possible that it was performed by earlier peoples. That the Jews did the operation successfully is shown by their laws. In the Mischnejoth (before 140 B.C.), the rights of twins delivered by section are gravely considered and in the Talmud (400 A.D.) the law reads, "a woman need not observe the usual days of purification after abdominal delivery." "Jotze Dofan" was the name they applied to a child delivered by operation through the flank of its mother, and "Kariyath Habbeten" to the classic cesarean. . . .[5]

The lack of information about cesareans extends from the pre-Christian era to the Renaissance period. *Gynecology and Obstetrics* reports:

> It will be seen, therefore, that the practice of obstetrics during the Renaissance remained much as it had been during the Greek and Roman periods with the result that, as Garrison puts it, "in normal labor, a woman had an even chance, if she did not succumb to puerperal [childbed] fever or eclampsia; in a difficult labor she was actually butchered to death by a Sairey Gamp [midwife] of the time or one of the vagabond "surgeons."[6]

The first successful cesarean section (successful in the sense that the woman lived through it) is recorded as having taken place in the year 1500. However, it was not noted until eighty-eight years later by Caspar Bauhin, so its veracity is subject to some debate. Factual or fictionalized, this first successful cesarean took place in Singerhausen, Switzerland, where Joseph Nufer, a castrator of pigs (swine gelder) performed the operation on his wife. The Nufer family must have had some means, or at least influence in the community, for it is said that thirteen midwives were in attendance for this labor, which was long, complicated, painful, and without progress. Several stone-cutters were also reported present, although what they were there for is unknown. Nufer obtained permission from the authorities to do a cesarean and invited the midwives to stay. All but two left. As a swine gelder, Mr. Nufer must have been aware, however crudely and unknowingly, that sharp instruments, cleanliness, neat incisions, and suturing were essential, because the baby was safely delivered. We are told that it lived to the age of seventy-seven and that the mother later gave birth vaginally to twins and delivered four more times after that.[7]

Other instances of cesarean section were recorded during the sixteenth century. This surgical delivery was then frequently accompanied by removal of the uterus (hysterectomy) which was deemed necessary to stanch the hemorrhaging. On the small chance that the woman survived, it's highly unlikely that she would have wanted another baby, so the hysterectomy was an extreme but possibly welcome form of birth control. The possibility of the mother's survival was taken into account along with the grim alternatives: certain death for both, or death of the fetus by craniotomy (puncture of the skull to collapse the head, thus making it possible to remove the fetus). Champions of the cesarean procedure were often called assassins because of the extraordinarily high mortality rate.[8]

> Among the outstanding events of the Renaissance was the development of cesarean section of the living woman, in the major European countries. The death rate of cesarean section at this time was almost 100 per cent. So it was quite a desperate

> procedure and attempted only on women who were moribund [at the point of death]. However well-intentioned the operator, the bereaved relatives always had the feeling that the unfortunate mother might have lived if she had been left alone. . . .[9]

Because of the high mortality rate, the operation was banned in Paris during the seventeenth century.

In his work "The Country Midwife's Opusculum on Vade Mecum," Percival Willughby (1597–1685) of England had this to say about cesarean section:

> It hath proved unfortunate to severall, under whose hands the women have perished, and it is not used in England.
> Dr. James Primrose holdeth it to bee a rash peece of work, and to do it on a living woman, a practice to be abhored.
> I therefore pass over it with silence, being unwilling to make a dreadful noise in the cares of women, or to embolden any in the works of cruelty.
> Yet let mee not leave women in their sufferings comfortless, without any hope of cure, for that I beleeve this dreadful operation may, without cutting the mother's side, and womb, bee better performed, and helped, by drawing the child, if it bee living, by the feet; if it be dead, by the crochet. . . .
> I therefore prefer the use of the hand before the crochet, or any other instruement whatsoever.[10]

The Italian Scipone Mercurio (1550–1595?) is credited with greatly improving the knowledge of obstetrics and is said to have revived interest in the procedure:

> It was his observations on cesarean sections in France [1571] that prompted him to study under Arantius at Bologna on his return to Italy. From him, he learned much of obstetrics that bears

directly on the problems of cesarean section, such as pelvic contractions. . . . He was, so far as known, the first to suggest the advisability of a cesarean operation on a living mother with a contracted pelvis. . . . His description of cesarean section is very long and detailed, but a model of clarity. . . . Suffice it to say that they used no anesthesia. . . . The patient was held by five strong men (or strong, courageous women) in a big canopied bed. The incision was outlined in ink first. The uterus was sponged out, as was the abdominal cavity. The abdominal wall was closed by interrupted sutures, the intestines carefully pushed away in the process. The postoperative treatment was the same as for any other form of surgery. He ends his discourse by saying, "This is enough about this new method of aiding difficult deliveries to help miserable patients."[11]

A Dutch surgeon and a contemporary of Rembrandt, Hendrik von Roonhuyze, also advocated cesarean section and produced a remarkable book in 1663 that contained detailed copperplate illustrations showing his method.[12]

The first successful American cesarean took place in Edom, Virginia, on January 14, 1794, when Dr. Jesse Bennet's wife was having a long and difficult labor. Dr. Bennet called in a consultant, Dr. Humphrey, whose opinion was that should a cesarean section be performed, it would most assuredly be fatal to the mother. Mrs. Bennet wished to at least save the life of her child (craniotomy being the alternative) and so insisted upon the cesarean in spite of the consultant's dire predictions.

Mrs. Bennet was placed on planks stretched across two barrels. She was held down by two black servants, while her sister-in-law held a lamp. The only anesthesia was a large dose of laudanum. Dr. Bennet performed the operation assisted, however condescendingly, by Dr. Humphrey. Not only did the mother survive the delivery by thirty-six years, but the child is said to have lived for seventy-seven years.[13]

Another successful early American cesarean delivery took place in 1827. This operation, performed by Dr. John L. Richmond, was done upon a kitchen table with a penknife. It is said that this mother fully recovered in twenty-four days.[14]

In 1879 Felkin reported witnessing a cesarean delivery in Africa. The mother was made drunk on banana wine. Then the doctor's hands and the mother's abdomen were covered with wine. According to Felkin, the accuracy and speed with which the African doctor performed the cesarean caused him to speculate that perhaps the procedure had been known by these people for centuries.[15]

In addition to nineteenth-century developments of anesthesia and antisepsis (both unknown previously), one of the greatest advances in the cesarean delivery came in 1882 when Max Sanger developed a technique to close the uterine incision with sutures. Prior to this innovation, the uterus was always removed. With the suturing technique, removal was no longer deemed necessary.[16]

Myths, folk ballads, and folk tales all relate stories of women whose birth experiences included agonizing pain and often resulted in the deaths of both mother and baby. Surgical delivery was used only as a last resort when all other methods, potions, and incantations failed. Chances of survival for the cesarean mother were slim. It is only in the past few decades that the cesarean operation has become a relatively safe procedure for both mother and child.

CHOICES TO EXPLORE:
A CHECKLIST

"If you don't know your
options, you don't have
any."
— From *A Good Birth, A
Safe Birth*[1]

Unless you are a cesarean parent or have taken
the time to listen to cesarean parents talk about their experiences, you may be unaware of the depth of trauma many of
them experience. After more than a decade of talking to and
corresponding with hundreds of couples across the country, I
am still shocked and dismayed to hear their stories, which are
rife with dissatisfaction. The variety of cesarean parents'
emotions and reactions is limited only by the number of
parents who confront cesarean delivery. However, in order to
ensure a better birth experience for yourself, be it by cesarean
or vaginally, the most important thing to remember is that you
must know your options if you are to take advantage of them.

To be sure, if you must have a cesarean, it is impossible to do
so without the assistance and skill of a medical team and
modern equipment. But to say "They are going to take the
baby," as many parents erroneously do, is defeatist. "They" are
not going to take your baby. You are going to have your baby
with their help. You have choices regarding when, how, and
where your baby will be born, as well as who will be with you
during the birth. It is never too late to try to make your wishes
known, although ideally you should start as early in your

pregnancy as possible to ensure that you will have the options you want. Just as power is knowledge, so, too, is planning your ideal birth experience in advance.

One of the first questions you will have if you are facing a second or third cesarean is, "Why can't I have a trial of labor and spontaneous vaginal delivery?" The answer, in most cases, is that you *can*. (For a discussion of this see Chapter 16). However, if you must have a cesarean, here are questions you will want to explore in order to know what your options are:

1. *When will hospital admission take place?* Can it be arranged for the morning of the birth? Can the mother have preoperative tests (such as blood work) done on an outpatient basis a day or two before delivery so she does not have to spend the night before in the hospital?

A few hospitals already schedule important tests and interviews prior to admission or a few hours before the scheduled delivery. Coming to the hospital a few hours before the baby is born may ensure a better night's rest for the mother and will make the event seem more like a birth and less like a routine surgical procedure. In terms of dollars and cents, it probably allows a better utilization of hospital resources and may save the couple (or their insurance company or the taxpayer) the cost of an unnecessary overnight stay. Objections may be (a) the mother may not show up at the hospital in time (barring fire, flash flood, hurricane, or tornado, this objection is invalid); (b) the mother's condition cannot be monitored the night before; (c) the mother may spend the night "on the town" instead of resting quietly; (d) the mother may cheat and eat something after midnight (even in hospitals, food and water are available to the mother who wishes to "sneak" them); (e) it will cause a logjam of paperwork and preoperative procedures; and (f) admission the day before delivery is traditional.

2. *What kind of prepping is done?* There is no reason medically to perform total preps which remove all hair from beneath the woman's breasts all the way around to her tailbone. A partial prep is now acceptable to the obstetric

community. Check in advance to make certain that the doctor who is attending you follows current medical trends and womens' preference.

3. *What types of medication are given?* What are their effects, and what procedures are performed? These points are crucial. The mother will want to know in advance what is being given to her and why, for this also affects her baby.

4. *Is there a choice of anesthesia?* Unless there are medical contraindications (which the doctor will explain to the mother) may she have a voice in this decision?

5. *Can the father be present for the birth?* Even where hospital policies allow fathers to be present, some doctors may object. What is your hospital's policy and what are your doctor's feelings about it?

6. *Can a mirror be used?* If you would like to have one so you can see the baby's birth, will your doctor or hospital provide it?

7. *Will the infant's condition be judged on an individual basis?* What is the policy at your hospital? Can you make arrangements for a pediatrician to examine your baby within a short time after birth? Even if the hospital has a routine of placing all cesarean babies under observation in the special care nursery for a twelve- or twenty-four-hour period, is it possible for you to hold your baby within a short time after birth?

8. *Will you be able to hold and nurse the baby in the delivery room?* It is possible to nurse a cesarean baby within minutes after birth on the delivery table, as is done with vaginal births. Will the hospital allow the mother to do this?

9. *Where is the baby care unit placed?* In the delivery room, is the baby-warmer crib located where the mother can see?

10. *Will someone bring the baby to you within seconds or minutes after birth for viewing, examination, and breast-feeding?*

11. *Can you request that the baby not be given*

supplemental feedings if you decide to breast-feed? What is the hospital policy? Are babies in the nursery routinely fed supplements?

12. *Does your hospital have rooming-in?* If so, how flexible is the policy? How soon is it possible for cesarean babies?

13. *When are visiting hours for fathers?* Is he considered a "visitor" and allowed to come to the hospital only for an hour or two a day, or is he thought of as an integral family member free to visit as he wishes?

14. *If the father cannot be with you for the birth, can a significant other (such as a mother, sister, special friend, or birth attendant) be with you?*

15. *Is there sibling visitation?* May your older children visit you in the hospital? If so, when?

16. *What classes are available in your area for cesarean parents?* If none, is it possible to enroll in part of the regular childbirth education series and receive supplemental instruction from the teacher? Failing that, will your obstetrician and/or a maternity nurse or midwife address your questions and supplement the information available?

17. *Are VBAC (vaginal birth after cesarean) classes available?* Is there a doctor and a hospital in your area where subsequent vaginal delivery—or at minimum, spontaneous labor—is encouraged? If not, why not?

18. *Have you truly prepared yourself for birth?* Do you have a written list of choices you'd like honored? Have you planned for any contingency? Is your husband and/or labor attendant as well as your doctor and, when need be, the hospital staff and administrators aware of what you want?

EDUCATION AND SUPPORT

SUPPORTING CESAREAN PARENTS

When should parents be told that the doctor is considering doing a cesarean? Can telling them too early make them give up hope and just consent to a cesarean? Probably not, providing that the parents are educated and informed. It is better to tell parents as far in advance as possible so that they can employ any one or a number of preventive measures that may overcome the need for surgical delivery, and/or so that they may seek a second opinion before granting permission. At least with advance warning and advance preparation, parents who end up with a cesarean will know that they have tried everything in their power to accomplish a vaginal delivery.

Ruth Allen, a registered nurse and childbirth educator, offers this advice to hospital staff:

> When laboring couples are told may influence their reactions. The general practice is to keep them in the dark as long as possible. Not telling them makes it easier on the staff, both doctors and nurses. Couples who don't know won't ask questions, express their feelings, or need a lot of time

and support. They are instead "good patients," even if unknowing ones. One father had been coaching and supporting his wife through a long labor, with lengthy contractions every two minutes. The staff knew that a cesarean was almost inevitable two or three hours in advance, but the parents were not told until the last minute. The husband said afterward that if he had known there was a time limit, he would not have felt so discouraged. All he could see was labor going on indefinitely.

If possible, tell the couple when they are together. Offer a brief explanation of why and a simple step-by-step outline of what is to take place. The couple may not take it all in, but they will appreciate your time. Let them ask questions and express their feelings to you. Except in cases of real emergencies, such as abruptio placenta, there is time to explain.

In rush cases [when the father cannot or chooses not to be present], tell the father you will send someone to explain as soon as possible. Above all, talk to the woman as you are caring for her. Allow the couple to be together while preparations are being made. If the couple are together, they can hold hands, ask questions, and talk and cry (if they feel like it) while the mother is being prepped and the catheter inserted. It is important for the staff to have a "You're okay" attitude toward the couple. Let them know that they are free to express their emotions and touch each other if they want to.

In the cesarean delivery room, it is important to emphasize the birth aspect. This is not just a routine procedure to the mother or father, if he is present. As doctors and nurses, let us keep in mind that this is not a tumor being removed. Any and all talk should include the parents. Especially if the father cannot be present, it is our responsibility to make the mother feel involved and comfortable. We can talk with her and rejoice when the baby is born. The mother needs this support. We must constantly reassure her that she is doing well, that the baby is fine.

It will make a difference to the mother if she is able to establish eye contact (at least briefly at frequent intervals) with her obstetrician. [And even better if she can establish eye contact with the baby's father or her support person.] The doctor may not have been trained to deal with emotions but only how to perform a technically perfect operation on an organ. When [the doctor] was trained, he may have dealt only with patients who were heavily medicated and given general anesthesia. Today's philosophy of using spinal or epidural anesthesia and as little medication as possible, coupled with the assertiveness of parents who want a human, warm experience is a totally different situation.[1]

Parents who tell or write their obstetricians, hospital administrators, and childbirth educators detailing what they did or did not like about their experiences (rather than becoming increasingly bitter and frustrated) will help the medical establishment realize what a positive difference they can make. This holds true too for those advocating better cesarean birth experiences, fewer cesareans, and trials of labor and subsequent vaginal deliveries as the *norm* now and in the future.

PREPARED CHILDBIRTH CLASSES

Should traditional prepared childbirth classes include information on the possibility of cesarean section? And if so, how much and what kind of information is appropriate? In my view, instructors should include adequate information on cesareans so that parents are prepared just in case. In addition, it is imperative to include information on how to prevent unnecessary cesareans. It is better to expect the best and be prepared for the worst.

Until the mid- and late-seventies, little or no information about cesareans was included in prepared childbirth classes. In the first edition of this book, I suggested that in order to truly prepare all couples for any eventuality, all prepared childbirth education courses should include more than brief mention of cesarean delivery. I continue to believe that no parent should have to face any form of birth unprepared.

Taking the ostrich approach by not discussing the subject of cesarean birth in today's preparation classes is unlikely to result in any benefit. Before most self-respecting childbirth educators included information on the subject approximately 20 percent of all births took place by cesarean. This was in part because too many parents who had taken prepared or natural childbirth classes still had to confront giving birth surgically with little or no understanding of how they might possibly avoid a cesarean. In addition, they were unprepared for how to cope when a cesarean was necessary. As a direct result, a majority of cesarean parents felt sad, angry, confused, and sometimes bitter. They blamed themselves, were convinced that they were failures, and felt guilty. Worse still, they felt cheated—and not just out of a vaginal birth. They felt cheated because their doctors, their childbirth educators, and their birth attendants failed to provide them with adequate information and support.

It is the responsibility of educators to instill in parents-to-be an understanding of just how serious a cesarean is. Parents must know about interventions and how and when and why they should be avoided. At the same time, it stands to reason that class instructors should include information on preoperative procedures, what happens during a cesarean, how long one takes, and how parents will feel emotionally and physically during and after the birth. Information on cesarean prevention should be emphasized throughout the class series, from the introductory class when the aims are discussed through classes on newborn care, just as information on what happens during a cesarean should continue to be part of the class curriculum. The reason for this is clear: even once the cesarean rate falls, there are always going to be a certain number of babies born in this manner.

No parent that I know of has ever chosen to have a cesarean just because it might be a good experience when vaginal delivery was irrefutably possible. Further, I know of no childbirth instructor who indoctrinates parents-to-be with the notion that cesarean delivery is preferable to vaginal delivery. We must be careful not to treat the subject of cesarean childbirth too casually, thus tacitly implying that parents-to-be should accept this intervention without first trying to avoid it, but we should also make it clear that some cesareans are inevitable and medically valid. Educators must help parents understand both how to prevent unnecessary cesareans *and* what to do should one take place. By providing adequate information, the educator will help make the emergency cesarean less of a catastrophe, less of a major trauma. As we all know, even the most highly motivated, enlightened, and assertive parents sometimes find themselves in the operating room when they give birth.

However, while I think we must continue to discuss unexpected cesareans, not enough emphasis has been given to the fact that most cesareans are avoidable, as are most interventions. It is to the detriment of all parents to be unaware that over the past decade, indications for interventions and cesarean sections have grown to encompass the most flimsy of pretexts.

Dr. Robert Mendelsohn, author of *Mal(e) Practice,* uses the euphemism "creative diagnosis" to describe doctors who keep themselves busy—and cesarean rooms full—by using the power of suggestion to induce problems where there were none before (conditions of this kind are known as "iatrogenic"). Are parents aware of this? They should be. As Dr. Mendelsohn and a host of authors, researchers, and consumer advocates have shown, medical school training inevitably concentrates on interventions and regards birth as a high-risk medical crisis, rather than a normal, natural process. Many doctors themselves contend that they are overtrained when it comes to childbirth. Yet many of these same honest physicians feel compelled to use what they have been taught in training, regardless of whether or not it is necessary, and irrespective of the fact that these zealous practices are often counterproductive to ensuring safe, normal births. This approach to childbirth, as Dr. Mendelsohn points out, is ". . . responsible for a whole catalogue of creative symptoms, most of them scarcely heard of twenty years ago. The diagnoses include fetal distress, failure to progress, arrested descent, failure to dilate, and God knows what else. Meanwhile prolonged labor has been redefined. The duration of [normal] labor taken as an indication for Caesarean section has dropped progressively from the seventy-two hours that was generally accepted when I began my medical practice. It dropped to forty-eight hours, then twenty-four hours, twelve hours, and now, if the doctor is eager enough, even two hours will do."[2]

Is sufficient childbirth class time being devoted to *discouraging* parents from accepting any and all medical interventions, drugs, and arbitrary time limits? Will parents leave classes knowing the benefits and risks of commonplace medical routines? Do they know that these interventions can lead, in and of themselves, to otherwise preventable problems and cesarean sections? Is the childbirth educator scrupulous and fair in informing parents of the benefits and risks of obstetrical rituals that are potentially harmful? Do childbirth education courses offer a list of alternatives in terms of doctors, nurse-midwives, labor attendants, *doulas* (a Spanish word meaning women who care for and support laboring and birthing women), monitresses (private woman nurses hired to give one-on-one professional attention and encouragement to the parents during their labor and delivery), Alternative Birth Centers, and other resources? Even if these options are not "mainstream" and/or officially approved by the educator or the method she teaches, they should be made known.

It is grossly unfair to place the burden of reducing the number of cesareans, opening up options for VBACs, and getting information regarding the benefits and risks of interventions exclusively on the shoulders of expectant parents and birth activists. This is and should be the responsibility of doctors and health care providers, not the consumers. Thus far, however, the majority of the medical establishment has done little to change the nature, thrust, and practices of modern obstetrics, so the changemakers are, primarily, from among the consumer population.

It is past time to take the crisis out of childbirth and to replace hasty, common interventions with more natural approaches. Childbirth has become a technological toyland. In a way, this is not surprising, since high technology has entered our homes, our work places, every aspect of our lives. We live in an era of home computers, microwave ovens, video recorders, Dolby stereo, laser disks, video arcades, and space shuttles. Unless informed that high tech in the labor and delivery rooms may carry risks and dangers, why should parents question it? After all, it is everywhere else. Many expectant parents turn to doctors, childbirth educators, and the advances of technology as simply the ways and means of accomplishing the goal of gestation: having a baby. They may consider interventions and technology unthreatening. In addition, many of today's health care consumers are no different from the conventional patients of yesterday. Parents-to-be may still place blind faith in their doctors and hospitals. Their reasoning is that these experts should know what they are doing. If this were a heart transplant, they would want and expect every possible modern intervention and methodology. Why, then, should childbearing be that much different?

How do parents reconcile the benefits of technology in other aspects of medicine with the risks it often brings to the birth of a baby? We must return birth to nature's usually more-than-competent hands, and this may mean the re-education of parents who come to classes. Sadly, it is not easy to convince expectant parents that they should seriously question—if not refuse outright—much of the advice of modern obstetrics. The point is this: the issues confronting childbirth today are different from those that were standard even a few years ago. In addition to all the usual information offered in childbirth classes, it is necessary to discuss why and how seemingly benign interventions into the normal birthing process can and often do promote an escalating series of even more interventions, including the ultimate intervention, cesarean section. It is important not only to address but to *stress* the risks inherent in many commonplace obstetrical practices. It is time to teach natural (and sometimes ridiculously simple) ways of over-coming and correcting so-called problems that may arise during pregnancy, labor, and delivery *before* intervention is employed. This means that the normal variations of pregnancy and birth need to be taught so that variations are not confused with complications.

Further, it is imperative to bolster parents' self-confidence. The benefits of positive thinking cannot be emphasized strongly enough. But how do childbirth educators foster the belief that having a baby is a normal, natural event and that in almost all instances it can and should take place without interventions, while at the same time helping cesarean parents? How do they teach the joys and benefits of natural birth without contradict-ing themselves and giving double messages to cesarean fam-ilies? How do they prepare parents for the possibility of a cesarean without being too negative or too positive? Educators do not want parents to become too frightened, nor do they want to make the experience sound so easy, low risk, and emotionally rewarding that parents become sitting ducks for interventions and unnecessary cesareans.

The answer, quite possibly, is for childbirth educators to

address *all* issues of contemporary childbirth. This includes enumeration of interventions, their risks and benefits, and how to cope with any event. As a result, parents who do require cesarean delivery will have the reassurance of knowing what to expect, how to cope, and how to do everything they possibly can to prevent surgical delivery. Once a cesarean has taken place, at least they will no longer blame themselves or feel that they were unwittingly manipulated.

A review of current literature as well as discussions with parents who have recently had their babies by cesarean show that educators must continue to provide adequate information on what to expect and how to deal with whatever problems arise. In fact, many parents report that they were well informed and well prepared (often by doing extra studying and reading outside the classroom). They feel they were able to make intelligent decisions regarding their pregnancies, labors, and deliveries. They are satisfied that they made the right choices and put to good use many of the prevention measures they learned. Although these parents did not accomplish their goal of having a vaginal birth, they do not feel that they were victims of needless surgery. One of the major responsibilities of the childbirth educator is making sure that parents know what their options are.

THE CESAREAN REVOLUTION

In the mid 1970s, when the cesarean birth movement began, the objective was to fill a gap. Never before had there been so many cesareans, and never before had anyone concerned themselves with what to do for parents who gave birth by cesarean. When Ruth Allen and I established the world's first classes in prepared cesarean childbirth, and when this book was first published, our intention never was to promote more cesareans. Our concern was how to help parents who gave birth by cesarean. These parents were often sad, angry, and confused. Until 1974, there was no literature for cesarean parents to read, no classes for them to attend, no organizations to offer peer support (C/SEC was then a fledgling organization), no recognition from any quarter that took into account their growing numbers and their specific needs.

Prior to the revolution, parents often had very bad experiences. Giving birth is, unquestionably, one of the most profound and significant events in the life of any couple. And if having a baby meant having it by cesarean, then consumers, individually and in groups, saw to it that at least couples were not made outcasts or denied the most positive birth experience possible under the circumstances. With our prepared cesarean childbirth classes, Ruth and I found that couples approached delivery with greater confidence, had smoother recoveries, and experienced many of the same happy emotions that vaginal-delivery families enjoyed. We lobbied to have fathers present during cesarean births. Mothers wanted to keep their babies with them, providing the babies were healthy, and we helped to change policies so that mothers could do so. Women wanted spinal or epidural anesthesia rather than general, which was quite common then, so they could be awake when their babies were delivered. Doctors eventually agreed that this was beneficial, and they started to administer these types of anesthesia for cesarean birth. Parents wanted rooming-in, breast-feeding support, family-centered care, and a host of other options. Finally, cesarean parents are now able to enjoy the same programs available to vaginal-delivery parents and babies.

Today, however, the time has come to almost entirely eliminate prepared cesarean childbirth classes. Instead, classes in *cesarean prevention* and how to accomplish vaginal delivery following one or more cesareans should be offered. Prepared cesarean childbirth classes should not be done away with entirely, since resources must still be made available to those parents who give birth by cesarean. As the cesarean prevention movement takes hold, however, prepared cesarean childbirth classes can be phased out with few exceptions.

For the benefit of childbirth education programs that encompass the needs of parents who must give birth by cesarean, the following class outline is suggested:

THE CESAREAN BIRTH METHOD

Class 1. Most couples will have pre-enrolled. Since this is now a class exclusively for mandatory cesarean parents, and because these parents are at high risk or have clear medical reasons why they are not candidates for subsequent vaginal delivery, even when the most liberal standards for VBAC are applied, it is important that the instructor be aware of the medical and emotional needs of each class participant. Because of their special circumstances, many of these parents will come to class with very high levels of anxiety. Instructors will have to spend additional time on the areas of interest and concern that make each couple's situation exceptional.

In prepared cesarean childbirth classes, it is especially important to devote much of the class discussions to encouraging parents to talk about prior birth experiences and to helping alleviate their fears and very real concerns about not undergoing normal pregnancies and deliveries. Talking about prior experiences and dispelling any myths parents bring to the pregnancy are important aspects of preparing these parents. Discussions of fetal growth and development, using visual aids, are more effective than dry, lengthy lectures on anatomy and physiology.

The mothers are going to experience many of the same discomforts of pregnancy as any other woman, and information on how to cope with and avoid or overcome the usual side effects of pregnancy will be useful. Teaching them how to relieve backache, heartburn, leg cramps, and so on is important.

Because of their special status, many of the women in the

class will undergo antenatal tests. When discussing amniocentesis, ultrasound, etc., the responsible instructor will talk about benefits as well as risks. No pregnant woman should submit to any of these tests without thorough understanding of their potential hazards. Except where medically mandated, even high-risk cesarean mothers should be encouraged to refuse all but the most essential interventions.

Encouraging good nutrition is timely no matter what stage of pregnancy mothers in the class have reached. (It is hoped that your community offers classes in early pregnancy as well as in the last trimester.) For women who must have a cesarean, good fetal outcome is enhanced by good nutrition. What's more, a well-nourished woman who gives birth operatively will probably feel better and recuperate faster.

Signs of labor and what to do are an important subject for two reasons: (1) unless there are compelling medical facts that rule out spontaneous labor for a few of these parents, their having to give birth by cesarean does not automatically preclude the majority from being eligible to await the onset of labor before the cesarean is performed; and (2) despite doctors' best efforts to circumvent nature, it is to be expected that even when the cesarean has been scheduled, some mothers' bodies are going to surprise everyone by going into labor in advance of manmade timetables.

It is important to explain the function of Braxton Hicks contractions, how to cope with them, and how to differentiate them from "the real thing."

Relaxation breathing techniques, the pelvic rock, and other prenatal exercises should be covered in class. Relaxation breathing will relieve tension and/or physical discomfort during spontaneous labor, prenatal tests, the delivery, the postpartum period, and internal examinations.

Class 1 is a good time to introduce abdominal tightening exercises to relieve gas pains after surgical delivery. These techniques should be reiterated throughout the series.

Class 2. The second class is the time to discuss everything from hospital admission and the attending paperwork to how to relieve stress or ennui and apprehension while waiting for the birth to commence. Admission to the hospital a few hours before the birth (with, of course, a few exceptions) is or should be possible for these parents. As has been traditional in these classes since their inception, much time should be devoted to reviewing preoperative routines, medications that may be offered preoperatively (and why to avoid them, when possible, and what effects drugs such as Valium and Nembutal may have on the baby), and how to make the administration of anesthesia easier and more comfortable. When the actual delivery is discussed, be frank about offering information on topics such as fundal pressure (see page 121), hypotension, and other side effects that may arise during cesarean delivery. Knowing what to expect and how to cope is imperative. The role of the father in the delivery room should encompass what he may feel, what he'll see, how he can offer his support to the mother, what he will be able to do after the baby is born (cuddle it, hand it to the mother, help her while she holds the baby and starts to breast-feed while the operation is completed), what will be done for the baby immediately after delivery, and what to expect should special care of the newborn be needed. Not every parent will have a good outcome. Some babies will be very sick when delivered and because of this, in this type of class, it would seem relevant to include information on special care and intensive care nurseries, what will be done for the baby, what parents can do if their babies are sent to a high-risk unit. It is not too soon, either, for parents to make decisions about what they will do if their baby must be transferred to a neonatal intensive care unit in a hospital other than the one in which the mother gave birth. This class is also the time to talk about the recovery room period, how the mother might feel, what she will and will not be able to do, which members of her family will be able to visit with her there, and how long she can probably expect to stay before being transferred to her room. As always, rehearse relaxation breathing and abdominal tightening.

Class 3. If classes are taught in a hospital, conduct a tour of the maternity floor, labor and delivery rooms, recovery room, and nurseries. If classes are offered elsewhere, see if you can arrange for your class to tour a local hospital. If not, offer a slide or videotape presentation that includes explanations of all equipment that might be used in the delivery room and nurseries. There are a number of slide presentations and films available on cesarean birth. At least one such audio-visual aid should be presented. If they have not already done so, parents should prepare a written list of "Birth Plans" or "Birth Requests" that they wish to have honored; the class can compare notes and add to or delete from their lists. Despite the fact that many of these mothers and/or their babies may be at high risk, emphasize the fact that many times their births will go smoothly and their babies will be perfectly fine. In the event that all does not go well, follow-up on behalf of the instructor will enable her to provide these parents with resources such as books and local organizations for grieving families. (One of the most helpful books I have read on the subject is *When Pregnancy Fails* by Susan Borg and Judith Lasker.) Closing the class with a discussion of Birth Requests lists is a provocative way to encourage parents to think about what they want and what options may be available to them that they may not have considered.

Class 4. This is the time for the postpartum discussion. Although information should, in the main, focus on parenting a healthy newborn, coping with a less-than-perfect outcome can also be discussed. Some parents may already have had tragic or near-tragic experiences with prior births and may share their feelings and coping measures. Otherwise, these parents need information on all the usual postpartum subjects, including infant care, breast-feeding, birth control, sexual readjustment, layette needs, touching and bonding, and caring for older siblings as well as a newborn.

For this class, invite two or three couples from prior classes to share their birth experiences and answer questions. Often the experiences of former class parents and how they coped are more meaningful and enlightening than the instructor's curriculum itself. The series of classes could end with a film on the postpartum experience. Diplomas and gift packs can be given out, followed by a party with refreshments supplied by the class members, which will end the classes on a festive and positive note.

Miscellaneous Notes on Classes. You may wish to invite an obstetrician or anesthesiologist to Class 3 to address parents' questions. This is optional and depends upon how beneficial you feel such a question-and-answer period would be to your class participants.

Relaxation breathing techniques should be practiced before the close of each class. Teaching cesarean mothers how to do Kegals (see p. 44) is also advised since Kegals are important for all women to do in order to keep the pelvic floor conditioned and perhaps prevent such conditions as a prolapsed uterus.

The father's participation is encouraged in all phases of the classes and hospital stay. Even when fathers are permitted to be present for cesarean delivery, not every man will want to be present. Nonetheless, there are many contributions he can make to the pregnancy, delivery, and postpartum periods.

Audio-visual aids are important. From our own class experience, Ruth and I have learned that detailed, graphic pictures that concentrate *only* on the surgical technique upset parents. Photographs or films made from an angle where the mother is shown as the physicians operate are much more reassuring. Cesarean parents have expressed distaste when shown photos and films that are more appropriate as teaching aids for doctors and nurses in training. Slides and films should emphasize the birth aspect as well as some of the basic operative procedures. You may want to prepare your own slides, videos, or films in place of or to supplement other audiovisuals available through a variety of sources.

When the father cannot or refuses to attend classes, by all means let the mother know that she is welcome to invite a sister, friend, or her mother to come to classes and share the delivery in the father's stead. In some classes, instructors welcome fathers *and* a significant other as well as a labor attendant.

Observers such as student nurses or instructors-in-training are welcome, provided they are unobtrusive and few in number. The integrity of the couple's relationship with their childbirth educator must be maintained. Too many observers may make parents feel like guinea pigs and may inhibit them from speaking up and sharing their feelings.

When parents-to-be who must give birth by cesarean attend prepared childbirth classes; read as many books as they can on pregnancy, delivery, and the postpartum period; and share past experiences and hopes for this delivery, they have a greater understanding, a wider perspective, and an enhanced sense of security. Knowing what to expect, how to cope, and what other parents share in common with them enables cesarean parents to be more relaxed and enjoy their births to the fullest.

SUBSEQUENT VAGINAL
DELIVERY: THE VBAC
OPTION

Although the birth rate has fallen over the past few decades, the obstetrical profession has concurrently transformed itself from one of the lowest-paid medical specialties into one of the highest paid. This is attributable, in large part, to the fact that doctors collect more money to perform a cesarean than they do to attend a vaginal delivery and, at the same time, charge additional fees for antenatal tests and other high-tech interventions. There is no economic incentive to dissuade doctors from performing cesareans, and they continue to do so in spite of the recommendations the National Institutes of Health published in 1980, which concluded that the cesarean rate is too high.[1] Worse still, the most recent statistics available show that the cesarean rate has continued to climb without exception throughout the United States.

In December of 1984, Dr. Norman Gleicher, who is head of the obstetrics and gynecology department of Mt. Sinai Medical Center in Chicago, published a study on the proliferation of cesareans in the prestigious *Journal of the American Medical Association (JAMA)*. Dr. Gleicher concluded that the proliferation has occurred because, first, doctors collect larger fees for cesareans than they do for vaginal deliveries, and second, because performing cesareans enables doctors to arrange their schedules more efficiently. A third factor is that many obstetricians are afraid they will be sued for malpractice if they do not perform a cesarean. These are the same three allegations birth activists (primarily lay persons, although a few professionals have spoken out despite pressure from their peers) have been making for at least the past decade. In addition, physicians and hospitals may tacitly conspire to perform excessive numbers of cesareans. There is no motivation for hospital administrators and physician review boards to put a stop to the escalating rate of cesareans, because a cesarean mother and baby remain in the hospital many days longer and incur many more incidental charges than a woman who has a vaginal delivery.

Dr. Gleicher is a well-respected member of the medical mainstream. He is not an "outsider" or a "radical dissident" or a "consumer activist." To prove this point, consider the fact that in 1982 Dr. Gleicher published an article in *JAMA* that dispelled the myth—commonly believed by consumer activists— that fewer cesareans were performed on weekends than during weekdays so as not to interrupt doctors' days off. Dr. Gleicher's 1982 study found this contention to be without merit, and said so in emphatic terms.

In his 1984 *JAMA* report, Dr. Gleicher compared cesarean rates from the year 1977 to just prior to publication of his report. He wanted to determine why the cesarean rate was rising even in face of warnings from within the medical community. His goal was to determine what effect the 1980 NIH study, performed by a national, blue-ribbon panel, had on obstetrics. The conclusion of the NIH study was, as noted, that obstetricians are performing far too many cesareans, and it recommended that subsequent vaginal delivery be implemented to replace routine repeat cesareans. The findings and recommendations of the NIH panel were widely publicized in both the lay press and professional journals. Even so, as Dr.

Gleicher added in a December 31, 1984, *Newsweek* interview, "the obstetrical fraternity apparently failed to take note."

In 1981 Dr. Robert Mendelsohn offered this on the subject of change within the medical establishment:

> The National Institutes of Health (NIH) shot down the long-held obstetrical concept that once a woman has given birth by Caesarean section, all subsequent babies must be delivered in the same hazardous way. . . . I won't deny that I am mildly encouraged by the AMA . . . the NIH, the ACOG, and the FDA. . . . But rhetoric isn't reality. Until I see convincing, sustained evidence that doctors are practicing what their leaders are preaching, I'm not going to put my mirror [so that doctors could look at themselves] away.[2]

Dr. Mendelsohn's observations were nothing short of prophetic, in light of Dr. Gleicher's 1984 findings. One would have assumed that the 1980 NIH recommendations would have been followed by practicing physicians. They have not. Or at least they have not been on a large scale thus far.

In January 1982, the American College of Obstetrics and Gynecology (ACOG) issued a committee statement entitled, "Guidelines for Vaginal Birth After a Previous Cesarean Birth." This statement was revised in November 1984.[3] To this day, however, if you want to avoid a repeat cesarean and find a doctor and hospital who support vaginal birth after one or more cesareans, chances are you may have difficulty. The cesarean rate at this point shows no signs of dramatic decline. In fact, the most recent statistics available from across the United States tell us that the incidence continues to escalate. Here are some statistics on the increase in the cesarean rate over the past seven years, taken from Dr. Gleicher's 1984 compilation:

> Los Angeles County: up from 15% to 17%
> Illinois: up from 14% to 18%

New York City: up from 19% to 22%
New York State: up from 14% to 19%
Washington, D.C: up from 19% to a staggering
   27%
Boston: up from 19.5% to 22.6%
Atlanta: up from 10.7% to 17.8%
Virginia: up from 9.3% to 15%

What these figures show is that although consumers have been calling for a reduction in the number of cesareans for years, and now even with the backing of the mainstream medical establishment, the rate of cesarean sections has continued to increase.

Parents who want vaginal birth after cesarean (VBAC) must today go to great lengths—and sometimes great geographic distance—in order to get it. Consider the example of Donald and Dellann Boland, a Santa Monica, California, couple, whose experience was reported in *The Clarion*, in an article entitled "Birth with a French Accent."[4] The couple had had a cesarean delivery in 1982 with a breech baby who died of "unexplained causes in an intensive care unit of a major university hospital at a cost of $120,000." For their next birth, the Bolands were unable to find anyone in the Los Angeles area who would support their desire for a subsequent vaginal delivery. As a result, the Bolands,

welcomed their daughter, Alice, into the world on May 10, 1984, in Pithiviers, France. Dr. Michel Odent, the internationally famous surgeon and Director of Obstetrics at the Central Hospital of Pithiviers, attended the birth. Alice was in a "footling" or "complete" breech position but was born without any medication or technological intervention while Mrs. Boland remained in a vertical squatting position. The actual delivery took about 30 seconds after a labor of under 45 minutes. . . . In Pithiviers Dr. Odent and his staff of midwives and assistants are able to handle the individual needs of

mothers and babies. Fathers stay in private rooms
together with them. Babies never stay in a separate
nursery. A large meeting room with a piano is used
for gatherings of parents with newborn children
and prospective parents who come to Pithiviers.
The community of Pithiviers does everything to
welcome future parents who arrive for the births of
their children.

Incidentally, whereas such individualized care and housing for
fathers within the facilities sounds expensive the total bill for
the Bolands came to $850.

Compare the Boland's VBAC with a French accent to the
guidelines issued by ACOG, which begins with this introduction:[5]

Of the more than 3.5 million babies born each year
in the United States approximately 20% are delivered by cesarean birth and, at present, approximately 40% of these cesarean deliveries are repeat
procedures. Although for many years physicians in
Western Europe have not regarded a previous low
transverse uterine incision as a contraindication to
subsequent labor and vaginal delivery, in most
instances this practice has not been followed in the
United States.

In 1980, the National Institute of Child Health
and Human Development Conference on Childbirth, after reviewing available data, concluded that
vaginal birth after cesarean birth is an appropriate
option. More recent data show that 50–80% of
patients with low transverse uterine scars who
attempt to deliver vaginally have successful vaginal
births. Data also show that maternal and perinatal
mortality rates with subsequent vaginal delivery are
no higher than those for repeat cesarean births.

Thus far, the ACOG guidelines appear (and, in fact, are)
quite revolutionary for this bastion of the American obstetrical

establishment. They seem to offer an unequivocal mandate for VBAC. However, read on:

> Although uterine rupture can occur, it is rarely catastrophic with the availability of modern fetal monitoring, anesthesia, and obstetric support services. The benefits of successful vaginal delivery include elimination of operative and postoperative complications and shortened hospital stay. Thus, a trial of labor after a prior cesarean birth is appropriate if adequate facilities and staff are available and there are no medical contraindications. Because risk of labor has not been assessed for patients with more than one prior cesarean birth, with a low vertical uterine scar, or with breech presentation, the guidelines *do not apply to these situations* [my emphasis].
>
> Following are suggested guidelines for those physicians and hospitals wishing to offer patients the option to attempt vaginal delivery after a prior cesarean birth:
>
> 1. The woman and her physician should discuss fully, early in the prenatal course, the option of a trial of labor. This would allow for discussion throughout the pregnancy to make certain the patient is aware of the benefits and potential risks.
>
> 2. Absolute cephalopelvic disproportion, although rare, remains a contraindication to a trial of labor. However, studies show that subsequent trials of labor are successful in up to 70% of patients in whom the indication for cesarean delivery was "failure to progress in labor."
>
> 3. A previous classical uterine incision remains a contraindication to labor.
>
> 4. There should be only one fetus and the estimated fetal weight should be less than 4000 g.
>
> 5. There should be continuous electronic fetal heart rate and uterine activity monitoring throughout labor, as well as staff and facilities required to respond to acute obstetric emergencies. . . .

Continuous electronic fetal monitoring and 24-hour blood banking capabilities should be available. . . . A physician who is capable of evaluating labor and performing a cesarean delivery should be immediately available. If an emergency cesarean delivery becomes indicated, professional and institutional resources must have the capability to respond to acute intrapartum obstetric emergencies such as performing a cesarean delivery within 30 minutes from the time the decision is made until the surgical procedure is begun.

Critics of the newest ACOG guidelines fear that the recommendations are not liberal enough. As they now stand, they rule out subsequent vaginal delivery for women who have had more than one cesarean. They also delete from the list of VBAC candidates women who are expecting twins or breech births, those who have had classic uterine incisions, and those who are expecting babies anticipated to weigh more than eight or nine pounds. Worse still, the guidelines at this time mandate routine, continuous fetal monitoring throughout labor. In order to accomplish continuous fetal monitoring, the amniotic sac (membranes) will probably be ruptured artificially. This will almost inevitably result in more repeat cesareans, not fewer. And although the ACOG recommendations do not explicitly state it, chances are good that in addition to routine, continuous fetal monitoring, there will be the full array of traditional hospital interventions that inhibit women from taking control (e.g., IVs, denial of nourishment by mouth, etc.). These interventions will contribute tangentially, if not directly, to more cesareans. They are, in essence, counterproductive to the goal of achieving more vaginal births after cesarean.

It may take time before many doctors and hospitals bring about changes favoring subsequent vaginal delivery. Medicine and obstetrics have made great strides since the early part of this century. Yet American doctors, unlike their European peers, have stubbornly held fast to the slogan coined in 1916 by Dr. Cragin, "Once a cesarean, always a cesarean." Until the past few years, our doctors openly embraced technology, innovations, and interventions while steadfastly continuing to allow their practice to be dominated by this vestige from another era. Meanwhile, doctors and midwives in Europe were successfully seeing at least 75 to 88 percent of their patients through vaginal delivery after cesarean. If subsequent vaginal delivery were not safe, then the practice would have been abandoned long ago.

Not enough can be said to dispel the myth that subsequent vaginal delivery is riskier than repeat cesareans. I stress this for the benefit of parents who may now be undecided about going forward with plans for a VBAC, or who are discouraged in their endeavors to find a doctor within reasonable distance who is supportive of this alternative.

Perhaps you are going to a doctor who encourages subsequent vaginal delivery, but you are the one who is not sure you want to go through with it. You may be more afraid of a vaginal delivery than of another cesarean. You may be one of the women who admits that you would rather face the risks of surgery than confront the pain and uncertainty of normal labor and delivery. But consider the following partial list of surgical risks:

> The mortality rate for cesarean mothers "is two to four times higher than for vaginal births . . . at least half of maternal deaths during cesarean section are caused by the operation itself—and are not simply the result of the mother's being in poor health."[6]
>
> Even if you are well nourished, do not smoke cigarettes or marijuana or take drugs, exercise regularly, and are otherwise a healthy pregnant woman, bear in mind that the side effects of

surgical delivery include, among others, scar infections (uterine and skin), organ perforations during surgery, frequent and often persistent bladder infections, fever, staph infections, and hemorrhage. If hemorrhage is severe enough, a hysterectomy will follow.

Postcesarean/postsurgical complications arise in 20 to 25 percent of all cesareans. Most of these result from infection. In addition, there is also the risk inherent in anesthesia. The risks of anesthesia include aspiration of vomitus, embolism, even death.

Mothers are not the only ones at risk from anesthesia and preoperative medications. Newborns can also be adversely affected by a depression of their body systems. It can result in breathing difficulties, jaundice, circulatory problems, inhibited sucking reflex, neurological impairment (which may evidence itself immediately or which may not show up until fifteen to twenty years later), and even neonatal death.

In addition to other risks to babies born by cesarean, and taking into consideration the fact that in a few cases a cesarean may save a baby's life, a 1979 report in the *American Journal of Obstetrics and Gynecology* has shown that the United States continues to have one of the highest newborn death rates of all developed nations in the world. In other words, the proliferation of cesareans has not resulted in fewer dead (or damaged) babies after all. This, however, is what doctors promised us would come about.

Consenting to an unnecessary cesarean means that you are subjecting yourself and your baby to greater risk, pain, debilita tion, and complications. You would not subject yourself to a kidney transplant unless you needed it. Why subject yourself and your baby to major surgery when you probably do not need a cesarean?

There is no question that when a cesarean is medically mandated, it can be a lifesaving and relatively safe technique to protect mothers and babies. There also appears to be a consensus that an incidence of approximately 5 to 10 percent is sufficient to cover contingencies that require surgical intervention. There is mounting pressure to normalize birth and, concurrently, reduce the number of cesareans. Slow progress by professional health care providers has been frustrating. Consumers are growing impatient, and they have every right to be. Vaginal delivery after cesarean is safer than repeat cesarean in almost all instances. Why, then, is the medical profession dilatory in providing this option universally?

Waiting for changes to come internally, that is, from within the medical profession itself, has been up to this point futile and disconcerting. If you are committed to having a safe birth, especially if it is a VBAC, then you are going to have to be a well-informed, assertive consumer, a change-maker. You may have to write letters to doctors, hospital administrators, obstetrical nursing supervisors, local papers, national magazines, and television stations. You will want to join groups such as CPM (Cesarean Prevention Movement), ICEA (International Childbirth Education Association), and so forth. (For a complete list of organizations, see Resources). While being critical, also remember to offer encouragement and support to pioneering doctors, midwives, and hospitals, who are already providing normal, natural births, subsequent vaginal delivery, and other options despite resistance among their peers. You will want to attend or work toward establishing VBAC classes and VBAC support groups. (For effective ways to be an assertive, effective consumer, an excellent source is *A Good Birth, A Safe Birth* by Diana Korte and Roberta Scaer.)

VBAC CLASSES

VBAC classes are currently available in some areas. If you are interested in establishing VBAC classes, Esther Booth Zorn, founder of the Cesarean Prevention Movement (CPM), and her staff of co-workers and advisors have prepared and made available a curriculum for their organization's VBAC classes. In addition to training childbirth educators, CPM is preparing self-study modules to be compiled in a loose-leaf notebook for easy updating. There is a growing demand for CPM's materials and programs. Each module will be supplemented by audio-visual aids. At present the CPM curriculum for childbirth educators and self-study include:

> Module I: Expressing feelings relating to present and past birth experiences
>
> Module II: Philosophies of childbirth and uterine dependability
>
> Module III: Physical and psychological interventions
>
> Module IV: Nutrition, exercise, and the issue of informed consent
>
> Module V: Drugs in pregnancy, labor, and birth
>
> Module VI: Choosing a medical team, planning your birth (birth environment, hospital request list for an ideal birth), medical records—fact or fiction, and variations and complications (posterior labors, emergencies, breech, multiple pregnancy)
>
> Module VII: The labor process (concepts of healthy pain, letting go, sexuality, vocalization)
>
> Module VIII: Grieving and healing
>
> Module IX: Psycho-physiological interactions (beliefs and attitudes that may or may not be conducive to positive birthing, affirmations for healing and a birth visualization)

Module X: Problem cards: general question and answer period.

The title for CPM's program is "Birth Works." To obtain more information or to order Birth Works Modules, write to The Cesarean Prevention Movement at its national headquarters, P.O. Box 152, Syracuse, New York 13210.

UTERINE DEPENDABILITY

American doctors persisted for years in their refusal to consider vaginal delivery for women who had had one or more cesareans and cited their fear of uterine rupture as their reason. This professional phobia was unfounded; they knew from their textbooks, their training, and their empirical observations that the risk of a uterine rupture is less than 1 percent. Yet women who protested the "once a cesarean, always a cesarean" adage were most often told by their obstetricians to find another doctor. Not surprisingly, even the most diligent search for a doctor within a hundred-mile radius who would attend a labor and vaginal delivery for a woman who had previously had a cesarean (or other uterine surgery) resulted in failure. Doctors continued to tacitly spread the myth that uterine rupture was always a catastrophe and would leave only about four minutes in which to get the baby out alive.

Such devastating events are almost never encountered. If a uterus is going to come apart, what will occur is not a ripping or explosion but rather a nonthreatening thinning of the uterine wall (called a "window") or a slight separation of the edges previously joined (this is called "dehiscence"). In their book *Silent Knife,* Nancy Wainer Cohen and Lois J. Estner support the contention that VBACs are safe by stating, "In the rare circumstances that a uterus with a previous cesarean does separate, the incision generally opens gently and neatly, like a seam or zipper. *We found no reports of maternal death associated with the lower segment incision in all the studies we surveyed; the incidence of fetal death associated with VBAC is agreed to be less than with elective repeat cesarean even by the most reluctant VBAC skeptics.*"[7] It is also interesting to note that if rupture of a classical uterine incision (which only about .5 percent of all cesarean mothers have) is to occur at all, it is more likely to take place during the last ten to fourteen days of pregnancy, not during labor, as we have been lead to believe. Further, uterine rupture can occur in women who have never had any type of uterine surgery and who are pregnant for the first time. In such cases, uterine rupture seems directly related to poor nutrition and low socioeconomic status.

Most cesarean mothers are not in danger of uterine rupture during subsequent vaginal delivery. For this reason, use of the term "uterine dependability" is encouraged in place of the incorrect and negative term "uterine rupture." One cesarean mother who successfully accomplished a VBAC made some valid and provocative points regarding subsequent vaginal delivery:

> I had no fear whatsoever that my scar would rupture with a VBAC. The doctor I went to for the cesarean is the head of one of the most prestigious medical schools in the country. He's also the author of several obstetrical textbooks and many widely-quoted journal articles. If he can't sew a uterus together securely, then no one can. Doctors who vehemently oppose VBACs even for women they've sewn up with their own two hands don't have as much faith in their own abilities as I do. This is utterly ridiculous and unnecessary. Even though I'm far more leery of doctors than I once was, I still believe most doctors are competent enough to put sutures in a uterus so that it won't rip open with a vaginal birth later on.

The fact that VBAC is a safe and preferable option may increasingly be more widely acknowledged, but having VBAC is still often difficult to accomplish. Finding the right doctor or midwife and the environment in which you feel most comfortable and secure can be a time-consuming, frustrating experience. A successful VBAC, whether it takes place in a hospital, birth center, or at home, requires greater effort on the part of the birthing mother and her mate than going forward with a repeat cesarean. You must be well prepared to meet with resistance and refuse to take no for an answer if you are turned away time and time again as you search for people and places that support your choice. You may, on the other hand, be fortunate enough to live in an area where you have easy access to compatible resources. If not, and your independent research fails to turn up any promising leads, by all means immediately contact friends, CPM, and C/SEC members, the La Leche League, the International Childbirth Education Association (ICEA), local childbirth educators and hospital personnel, and any other sources that may be able to provide you with the names of doctors and midwives who practice VBAC (see Resources). Follow up on any and all leads.

Above all, do not become discouraged. In every issue of *The Clarion* (published by CPM), for example, there are letters from VBAC parents that tell of individual quests to overcome what seemed to be impossible odds but which resulted, thanks to these parents' relentless efforts, in happy endings. For Esther Booth Zorn, having her daughter, Katie, by VBAC became the motivation for formation of the international Cesarean Prevention Movement. Regarding the overall VBAC issue, and specifically her own experience, she writes:

> "We did it!" is an often heard cry of VBAC parents. . . . We need to congratulate ourselves for the energy that we have put out in order to make changes in the birthing picture for today's women. We can gain further energy and courage to go on if we can see how far we have come already. . . .

It is fitting, at a time when we are enjoying a growing membership and increasingly supportive national attention, including newspaper stories in the *Wall Street Journal, Los Angeles Times, USA Today,* and many others, that the CPM logo . . . is what it is: a woman standing tall with pride as she carries her newborn beneath the arch of women's arms giving support. Behind her comes the throng of others who choose also to give birth on their own terms. This CPM woman, a cesarean mom, VBAC mom, or first-time mom, has made her choices and wishes to show others the way of individual responsibility, not system responsibility.

None of us is truly alone anymore. Feeling alone in our pain, disappointment, anger, sadness over our birth experiences made it so much harder to endure. But now the picture is changing as one by one we link . . . to make changes in the birthing image held by the "civilized" world.

While giving birth to Katie I pleaded for relief and asked one of my labor support people, "Can I do it?" To which the entire room of people responded, "You are doing it!" When it feels like the changes to be made are too big, too many, too impossible, remind yourself the changes are being made, you are doing it![8]

What motivates ordinary parents to opt for vaginal birth after cesarean, when obtaining this goal requires diligence and persistence above and beyond the norm? There are obviously many reasons for such tenacity and determination, but the issues for these parents center on the greater safety of a subsequent vaginal delivery, and the emotional and physical trauma inherent in cesarean section. This holds true even when the parents are able to enjoy all the benefits of Family-Centered Maternity Care. No matter how well the cesarean and ensuing hospital stay go, VBAC mothers and fathers often feel bruised and embittered because they were cheated out of a normal, natural birth, not out of true necessity, they often feel, but because of injudicious medical intervention.

Although each birth is unique, many issues common to parents who choose vaginal delivery after cesarean were highlighted in an interview with Carey and Marc Kaplan of Canoga Park, California, whose second son, Adam, had been born by VBAC just nine weeks earlier.

CAREY: When our first son, Bobby, was born five years ago, we attended Lamaze classes. The classes prepared us for what they might do to us in the hospital so that we wouldn't be scared when the doctors and nurses brought out all the machines and interventions. The classes didn't warn us to stay away from interventions, however.

MARC: The classes we took were not natural child-birth classes, they were prepared childbirth classes. And there's a difference.

CAREY: We took Bradley classes the next time, and they're called natural childbirth classes.

MARC: With Bobby the doctor told us that we might have to have a cesarean because he thought the baby was very large. He did an ultrasound and told Carey the baby was due in late August.

CAREY: I was expecting the baby in late August but he still hadn't been born in October. I was very eager to have my baby, obviously. Finally, on a Sunday in October, we went to the hospital at seven in the morning after quite a few bouts with false labor. I was three centimeters dilated when I got to the hospital. The doctor came in shortly after we arrived and informed me that he was going to pop my water. He didn't give me a choice; he just did it to make my labor go faster. He broke my membranes because he wanted me to have an internal fetal monitor right from the start of labor. He also had an IV put in. Marc became mesmerized by the monitor and watched it the whole time, rather than paying attention to me.

During labor I was checked internally every few minutes. I had so many hands up me, it was awful.

The doctor came back to the hospital about eight hours later. When he examined me, he said I was only five centimeters dilated. The nurse had just checked me a few minutes before the doctor came in and said I was eight centimeters. I don't know why there should be such a big disparity between her measurement and his. But the doctor got worried that I was only five centimeters and ordered an x-ray. The minute the doctor reviewed the x-rays, he said he had to do an emergency cesarean. But the operating room ws busy so we had to wait an hour. So much for an emergency cesarean! I had an epidural but I didn't think it was working so they gave me a Valium IV. I looked into the light over the operating table and saw the doctor cut me so I said, "Ouch!" I wish now that I had shut up because I wasn't in pain at all.

MARC: As soon as Carey said, "Ouch! You cut me," they put her out. But I got to stay. I sat down next to the anesthesiologist and started asking him what he was doing, what was going on. He was very personable, really nice. They cut Carey open quickly. Once they started, it was slash, slash.

I was holding Carey's hand and talking to her until they put her out. Then I just concentrated completely on the operation. I watched them pull Bobby's head out, suck out the mucus, and then pull him out all the way, and I found out we had a boy. They took the baby over and washed him up immediately. Then the baby and I went to the nursery. I got to hold him very briefly in the nursery. From there I went straight to Carey in the recovery room. Later that night, I got to hold the baby again, and Carey got to hold him for the first time—but only for a quick minute or two. We did get to do a little bonding, but not much.

CAREY: After the baby was born I joined a group in Santa Barbara for postpartum mothers. Half the women in the group had had cesareans. At the first meeting we were each asked to describe our birth experiences. Although I was very disappointed with the way mine had gone, because everyone else told such positive stories, when they got to me I told a positive story, too—even though that is not how I felt. I had to keep my feelings bottled up for years. My feelings kept building up so much that when I wanted to get pregnant a second time, it took me a year and a half just to conceive because I was so afraid of having another cesarean.

MARC: When Carey finally did get pregnant, we found a certified nurse-midwife who referred us to a doctor who did VBACs. But the obstetrician said that Carey was not a VBAC candidate because the charts she'd received from our first obstetrician listed the reasons for the cesarean as being CPD and borderline infant distress—whatever that is. Our former doctor had never even mentioned borderline fetal distress. We never called back or went to the new doctor again. For the next four months, Carey pretended she wasn't pregnant because she was so discouraged. When she was six months pregnant, I told Carey that we had to do something about getting a doctor fast.

CAREY: When Marc insisted that we needed to find medical help, I went to a local bookstore and found *How to Avoid a Cesarean Section* and *Silent Knife.* After I read those books, I decided that I was going to have a VBAC no matter what, and that what I really wanted to do was to have my baby at home. I did not want to go to a hospital and have an IV and a fetal monitor just because I was having a VBAC. I felt that if I did go to a hospital, it would just set me up for another cesarean. Through a network of friends, I obtained the names of several midwives and found one we liked, who liked us, and who was willing to do a VBAC at home. After that, I began to feel better, physically and emotionally.

MARC: The midwife told Carey that she was not getting enough protein because she hadn't taken care of herself during the first part of her pregnancy. So Carey increased her intake of protein because she wanted to be in top shape for labor and delivery.

When we decided to have the baby at home, we asked Bobby if he wanted to be there for the birth. Carey told him that it was bloody and that it would hurt her, but it wouldn't hurt the baby. He said he wanted to be there for the birth, but we reassured him that he could leave at any time. To prepare him fully, we took him to Bradley classes with us and Carey read lots of books to him. Bobby was fully prepared for it. We also had a friend of Carey's on standby to be our labor assistant.

CAREY: With this pregnancy I again had lots of false alarms before I actually went into labor. I lost my mucus plug a few days before Adam was born. The day he was born, I had been at the supermarket, when I felt something thick and gooey dripping down my legs. I started having contractions pretty regularly, too, so the woman at the check stand rushed me through. I called Marc, my labor assistant, and the midwife as soon as I got home. They all told me to wait an hour to be sure, then call them back. But before long, I just had to call Marc and ask him to come home right away because I was sure that this was the real thing. When the midwife arrived, she was really calm. I walked around our street a lot during labor, which was very relaxing for me. I did not feel as though I had to rush, or that I had to be somewhere under a lot of pressure as I would have had I gone to a hospital.

We also called our Bradley teacher because she was going to be there, too. This was her first VBAC at home. She'd attended VBACs before, but always in a hospital. And she'd attended a lot of home births, but never a VBAC before.

The midwife examined me and said, "I don't want to upset you, but your baby's breech." I'd seen the midwife just a few days before and the baby's head had been engaged then. I was shocked that the baby had turned in the meantime. I was also shocked when she told me I was already nine centimeters dilated. I just couldn't believe I was dilated that much because I was having such a good time. It was really easy. I was expecting to be only about five centimeters. When she told us that the baby was breech, she asked us if we wanted to go to the hospital, but Marc and I said no. Marc had asked her when we first started going to her how many breeches she'd delivered and she said about two hundred, so we felt totally confident that our midwife could deliver our baby successfully.

MARC: Our midwife had worked in South America, where she had never been able to transport anybody to a hospital. There simply was nowhere to go, so she had to depend entirely on herself. And she said that in America, women don't die. They just don't, because American women are healthier, there are better medical facilities, and there's always a hospital nearby. She has had babies die on her—that couldn't be helped—but she's never lost a mother. She wasn't worried at all, which really helped us.

CAREY: Because we were really confident, it helped us stay in control. We were always in control this time, not like the last time when we went to a hospital.

MARC: Carey and I had agreed that I would be the one to catch the baby, but under the circumstances the midwife had to do it because it required a certain technique.

CAREY: My immediate reaction when she said the baby was breech was to ask our midwife if she could turn the baby, but she couldn't because the baby was so far down in the canal. She thinks it's more dangerous to turn a baby than to deliver it breech. At that point, I gave up hope of having a VBAC. But my fears lasted only a few moments because our midwife described step by step how she was going to deliver the baby. I walked around or stood just before the baby was born. When the baby was coming out, I semi-squatted which felt good.

MARC: We knew the baby was breech, but it came as a total surprise to all of us when one of the baby's feet started hanging down. The midwife kept trying to push it up since she didn't want to deliver a footling. She wanted to deliver the baby butt first so Carey wouldn't tear much. But our baby turned out to be a double footling breech. When the cord fell out and the water broke, our midwife had to get the baby out really quickly. The last five minutes were really intense.

CAREY: They were also very painful. I screamed a little but the actual delivery went really fast and I had only a small tear, which didn't need stitches. My pelvis was supposed to have been too small to deliver Bobby vaginally, and Adam turned out to weigh a whole pound more! Adam's head was also larger than Bobby's. Of course, my scar did not rupture and my recovery was so much quicker. Best of all was that I got to hold Adam immediately.

MARC: I loved the whole thing. During pregnancy, we weren't going to tell our parents that we were having a home birth until after the fact. But Carey's mother asked where we were going to deliver, so we told her. Of course, she objected. But Carey wrote her a long letter about why we felt it was better and safer to have the baby at home and sent her a copy of some of the books we'd read.

CAREY: A week later, my mom called me up and said that although she was still a little scared, she felt so much better now that she understood. What I had said in my letter was that everybody's been hearing only one side of the childbirth story for so long, that it's time to hear the other side. I told her that *Silent Knife* was extreme and that even I didn't agree with everything but that it proved that VBACs—even VBACs at home—are safe.

MARC: The cost of a hospital birth versus a home birth was not a factor in our decision, although the local hospital charges about ten thousand dollars for a cesarean. Midwives in our area charge between five hundred and a thousand.

CAREY: The reason we had a home birth was

because we wanted to. Although I wasn't for home births when we started, I am now. I felt so relaxed at home. I was in my own environment. We had a home birth because I just did not want to have another cesarean.

MARC: It's important to stress that we were not forced into a home birth. We absolutely did not want to go to a hospital. It was our decision. But to make sure we'd made the right decision, Carey went to the local hospital before Adam was born to make a comparison. After all our years of believing that doctors are gods and that their word is law, it was hard for us to abandon that concept. Neither of us thinks doctors are totally wrong. But in this situation, we went to the hospital for a tour and Carey actually got the shakes just from being there.

CAREY: After that I just knew I couldn't walk into a hospital to have my baby. It didn't feel like the right place to give birth. It's a place for sickness, not for celebration.

MARC: We can say we made a conscious choice, and a good one.

CAREY: We did make contingency plans in case I had to go to the hospital. And the only reason I would have gone would have been if I'd had placenta previa or cord prolapse. When the cord came out before Adam, we couldn't go to the hospital. There just wasn't enough time. But if my cord had been out when I was at the supermarket, I would have gone to the hospital under those circumstances.

MARC: If it had been necessary for Carey to go to the hospital, our contingency plans were that as soon as the baby was born, I'd check him out of the hospital AMA (against medical advice) right away. We decided that I'd take the baby home and feed it water for the first twenty-four hours. Then Carey would have signed out AMA after twenty-four hours and come home, too.

CAREY: Neither Marc nor I ever worried, not even for one minute, that the baby or I would die or that a catastrophe would occur. We never worried about uterine rupture. Ruptures aren't likely to take place. And if they do, they're usually just little windows. It doesn't mean instant death to the baby. That's totally false. Sure, I read all the horror stories, but I felt very, very safe. I felt very confident that enough other people had had VBACs that I could have one, too.

MARC: A VBAC at home isn't for everyone. But almost everyone should try for a VBAC, even if it's in a hospital.

CAREY: Less than a week after Adam was born, I was ready to have another baby again. I finally felt complete.

The majority of VBAC parents choose the hospital as the place where they feel safest and most comfortable. One father whose first child was delivered by cesarean and whose second and third babies were hospital VBACs stated his views on why they chose a hospital. "We felt," he said, and his wife agreed, "that we had a responsibility to ourselves and our babies to go to a hospital. It gave us a sense of security we would not have had at home." A VBAC mother elaborated on her choice of a hospital VBAC by saying,

> We were not at all worried about uterine rupture or other problems. We were lucky, I guess, because we were able to find a doctor whose practices and philosophies suited our needs perfectly. For us, there was a great sense of confidence in ourselves, which was enhanced by having a really great doctor and a hospital where we could have a VBAC without interventions. My birth went normally and naturally. There was no fetal monitoring, no IVs, no drugs, no pressure on us to accept the interventions of the traditional medical establishment. We had our VBAC in the alternative birth room and could not have had a better, more rewarding experience anywhere. It was clearly the right decision for us.

CONCLUSION:
THE WAY IT SHOULD BE

If you are among the estimated 5 percent of the childbearing population that is mandated to give birth by cesarean because of unavoidable and uncontrollable medical conditions, it is comforting to know that there exists a climate of concern for your very special and very different needs. This concern makes it possible to have a relatively safe and rewarding family-centered cesarean, which enhances your physical safety as well as your emotional well-being and which encourages bonding between you and your baby as well as bonding with other family members. This is the way it should be.

Childbirth is not the time to be complacent or passive. There is far too much at stake, particularly in view of the fact that thousands of unnecessary cesareans take place each year. I urge you to seriously question the reasons you are given for needing a cesarean. Maybe you do need one. If you do, make sure it will be as good an experience as possible for you and your family. Statistically and empirically, however, you stand a far greater chance of not needing a cesarean than you do of being among the small percentage of women who do. Medicine has given us a lot of ingenious inventions and bewildering nomenclature but these take our attention away from the real problems. In other words, we sometimes become distracted, intimidated, and overwhelmed. This is not the way it should be.

Of childbirth in general, noted author and educator Sheila Kitzinger eloquently describes the situation as follows:

> The experience of bearing a child is central to a woman's life. Years after the baby has been born she remembers acutely the details . . . and her feelings as the child was delivered. One can speak to any grandmother about birth and almost immediately she will begin to talk about her own labours. . . .
>
> When women have suffered in childbirth—have felt humiliated and degraded by pain, through being the passive instruments of physical processes they could not understand—it is not only they who are affected. They carry with them through their lives the memory of this experience and by their attitudes towards childbearing affect other women and men—not only their own daughters and sons, but many others with whom they come into contact. . . .
>
> But when a woman has her baby happily she spreads a different spirit—a mood of gladness rather than dread and horror. . . .
>
> It is this spirit of hope, this joy in birth as a fulfillment of a man and woman's love for each other, that should be the essence of childbirth. . . .
>
> It is childbirth with joy.[1]

You have a choice regarding where and how you have your baby. You have a choice regarding who will be with you for the birth. You have abundant choices in all aspects of childbirth. These choices are not always easy to learn about, nor are they likely to be readily available without effort on your part. It is your decision. You can effect change. What your childbirth experience will be is for you to decide.

RESOURCES/ORGANIZATIONS

Networking (i.e., establishing communications with others to share information), as well as supporting others with philosophies and goals similar to yours, is essential in our quest for better, safer births for all childbearing families. Following is a list of national and international organizations of great importance to cesarean and VBAC parents. When sending inquiries and asking for local chapters, it is a good idea to send a stamped, self-addressed envelope as a courtesy.

American Academy of Husband-Coached Childbirth (also known as The Bradley Method)
Box 5224
Sherman Oaks, CA 91413

American College of Home Obstetrics
644 North Michigan Avenue
Suite 600
Chicago, IL 60611

American Foundation for Maternal & Child Health
30 Beekman Place
New York, NY 10022

American Society for Psychoprophylaxis in Obstetrics (ASPO, also known as the Lamaze Method)
1411 K Street, N.W.
Washington, D.C. 20005

Association for Childbirth at Home, International
Box 1219
Cerritos, CA 90701

Cesarean Connection
Box 11
Westmount, IL 60559

The Cesarean Prevention Movement
Box 152
Syracuse, NY 13210

C/SEC (Cesareans/Support, Education, and Concern)
22 Forest Rd.
Framingham, MA 01701

International Childbirth Education Association (ICEA)
Box 20048
Minneapolis, MN 55420

La Leche League, International
9616 Minneapolis Ave.
Franklin Park, IL 60631

National Association of Parents & Professionals for Safe Alternatives in Childbirth (NAPSAC)
Box 267
Marble Hill, MO 63764

NOTES

Chapter 2. Indications: Why Me?
1. P. R. Myerscough, *Munro Kerr's Operative Obstetrics,* Tenth Edition (London: Baillière Tindall, 1982), pp. 70, 71, 88.
2. Christopher Norwood, *How to Avoid a Cesarean Section* (New York: Simon and Schuster, 1984), p. 135.
3. Ibid., pp. 143–44.
4. Helen Marieskind, "An Evaluation of Caesarean Section in the United States," U.S. Department of Health, Education, and Welfare, 1980.

Chapter 3. Pregnancy
1. Editors of *Consumer Reports, "The Medicine Show,"* rev. ed. (Mount Vernon, N.Y.: Consumer Union, 1971), pp. 184–85.
2. Catherine Milinaire, *Birth* (New York: Harmony, 1974), p. 51.

Chapter 5. Tests to Determine Fetal Maturity and Well-being
1. Jonathan Scher, M.D., and Carol Dix, *Will My Baby Be Normal? How to Make Sure* (New York: Dial, 1984).
2. Christopher Norwood, *How to Avoid a Cesarean Section* (New York: Simon and Schuster, 1984), pp. 181–82.

3. Gail Brewer, *What Every Pregnant Woman Should Know* (New York: Random House, 1977), and Brewer and Janice Presser Greene, *Right from the Start* (Emmaus, Pa.: Rodale, 1981).

Chapter 6. Signs of Labor and What to Do

1. American College of Obstetrics and Gynecology, "Guidelines for Vaginal Delivery after a Previous Cesarean Birth," Committee Statement, January 1982, revised November 1984.
2. Robert S. Mendelsohn, M.D., *Mal(e) Practice* (Chicago: Contemporary, 1981), p. 182.

Chapter 8. Birthday!

1. "Rx for a Crisis," *Time,* June 16, 1975, p. 49.
2. Letter dated February 6, 1976, from J. Robert McTammany, M.D., of Reading, Pennsylvania, to the author.

Chapter 12. Human Bonding

1. Ashley Montague, *Touching* (New York: Perennial Library, Harper and Row, 1972; copyright 1971, Columbia University Press), pp. 65, 75–78, *passim.*
2. Ibid., pp. 91, 95, 138, *passim.*
3. Ibid., p. 53.

Chapter 13. History and Evolution of the Cesarean Delivery

1. Louis M. Hellman and Jack A. Pritchard, *Williams Obstetrics,* 14th ed. (New York: Appleton-Century-Crofts, 1971), p. 1164.
2. Nicholson J. Eastman and Louis M. Hellman, *Williams Obstetrics,* 12th ed. (New York: Appleton-Century-Crofts, 1961), p. 1179.
3. Joseph B. De Lee, M.D., and J. P. Greenhill, M.D., *Principles and Practice of Obstetrics,* 8th ed. (Philadelphia and London: W. B. Saunders, 1943), p. 1011.
4. Edwin M. Jameson, M.D., *Gynecology and Obstetrics* (New York: Hafner, 1962), p. 25.
5. De Lee and Greenhill, op. cit., p. 1011.
6. Jameson, op. cit., p. 41.
7. Theodore Cianfrani, M.D., *A Short History of Obstetrics*

and Gynecology (Springfield, Ill.: Charles C. Thomas, 1960), pp. 359–61.

8. Ibid., p. 361.
9. Cianfrani, op. cit., p. 131.
10. I. G. Cloud, M.D., "Cesarean Section on the Dead and Moribund," *Journal of the American College of Obstetricians and Gynecologists* (July 1960): 30.
11. Cianfrani, op. cit., pp. 150–51.
12. Ibid., p. 171.
13. Ibid., p. 264 (with additional details from a letter dated March 18, 1976, from Vance Watt, M.D., of Thomasville, Georgia, to the author).
14. Ibid., p. 361.
15. De Lee and Greenhill, op. cit., p. 1011.
16. Harold Speert, M.D., *Obstetric and Gynecologic Milestones* (New York: Macmillan, 1958), p. 594.

Chapter 14. Choices to Explore: A Checklist
1. Diana Korte and Roberta Scaer, *A Good Birth, A Safe Birth* (New York, Bantam, 1984), p. 33.

Chapter 15. Education and Support
1. Extemporaneous remarks based on an article by Bernie Donovan and Ruth Allen, *NAACOG Journal,* November/December 1977, pp. 37–48.
2. Robert S. Mendelsohn, *Mal(e) Practice* (Chicago: Contemporary, 1981), pp. 7–9.

Chapter 16. Subsequent Vaginal Delivery: The VBAC Option
1. Helen Marieskind, "An Evaluation of Cesarean Section in the United States," U.S. Department of Health, Education and Welfare, 1980.
2. Robert S. Mendelsohn, *Mal(e) Practice* (Chicago: Contemporary, 1981), pp. 7–9.
3. American College of Obstetrics and Gynecology, "Guidelines for Vaginal Delivery after a Previous Cesarean Birth," Committee Statement, January 1982, revised November 1984.

4. "Birth with a French Accent," *The Clarion* 2, no. 4 (1984): 1.
5. American College of Obstetrics and Gynecology, op. cit.
6. Christopher Norwood, *How to Avoid a Cesarean Section* (New York: Simon and Schuster, 1984), p. 168.
7. Nancy Wainer Cohen and Lois J. Estner, *Silent Knife* (South Hadley, Mass.: Bergin and Garvey, 1983), p. 84.
8. Editorial, *The Clarion* 3, no. 2 (1984): 1.

Conclusion: The Way It Should Be

1. Sheila Kitzinger, *The Experience of Childbirth* (Baltimore: Penguin, 1962–1972), pp. 17–18.

SUGGESTED READING

Arms, Suzanne. *Immaculate Deception: A New Look at Women and Childbirth.* South Hadley, Mass.: Bergin & Garvey, 1984.

Ashford, Janet I. *The Whole Birth Catalog: A Sourcebook for Choices in Childbirth.* Trumansburg, Pa.: Crossing Press, 1983.

Beals, Peg, ed. *ICEA Parents' Guide to the Childbearing Years.* Minneapolis: International Childbirth, 1980.

Borg, Susan, and Judith Lasker. *When Pregnancy Fails: Families Coping with Miscarriage, Stillbirth, and Infant Death.* Boston: Beacon Press, 1981.

Boston Women's Health Cook Collective. *The New Our Bodies, Ourselves.* New York: Simon and Schuster, 1985.

Brewer, Gail S., and Janice P. Greene. *Right from the Start: Meeting the Challenges of Mothering Your Unborn and Newborn Baby.* Emmaus, Pa.: Rodale Press, 1981.

Cohen, Nancy Wainer, and Lois J. Estner. *Silent Knife: Cesarean Prevention and Vaginal Birth after Cesarean.* South Hadley, Mass.: Bergin & Garvey, 1983.

Davis, Adelle. *Let's Get Well.* New York: New American Library, 1972.

―――. *Let's Have Healthy Children.* Rev. ed. New York: New American Library, 1981.

Duffy, Cynthia L., and Linda Meyer. *Responsible Childbirth:*

How to Give Birth Normally and Avoid a Cesarean Section. Saratoga, Calif.: R & E Pubs., 1984.

Elkins, Valmai H. *The Rights of the Pregnant Parent.* New York: Schocken Books, 1980.

Gaskin, Ina May. *Spiritual Midwifery.* Rev. ed. Summertown, Tenn.: Book Publishing Co., 1978.

Haire, Doris. *The Cultural Warping of Childbirth.* (Available through ICEA.)

Kitzinger, Sheila. *The Experience of Childbirth.* 5th ed. New York: Penguin, 1984.

Klaus, Marshall H., and John H. Kennell. *Parent-Infant Bonding.* 2nd. ed. St. Louis: Mosby, 1982.

Korte, Diane, and Robert Scaer. *A Good Birth: A Safe Birth.* New York: Bantam, 1984.

Mendelsohn, Robert S. *Male Practice: How Doctors Manipulate Women.* Chicago: Contemporary Books, 1981.

Milinaire, Catherine. *Birth.* Edited by Joseph Berger. New York: Crown, 1974.

Mitchell, Kathleen, and Marty Nason. *Cesarean Birth: A Couple's Guide for Decision and Preparation.* New York: Kampmann, 1981.

Noble, Elizabeth. *Essential Exercises for the Childbearing Years.* Rev. ed. Boston: Houghton Mifflin, 1982.

Norwood, Christopher. *How to Avoid a Cesarean Section.* New York: Simon & Schuster, 1984.

Odent, Michel. *Birth Reborn.* New York: Pantheon, 1984.

Panuthos, Claudia, and Catherine Romeo. *Ended Beginnings: Healing Childbearing Losses.* South Hadley, Mass.: Bergin & Garvey, 1984.

Panuthos, Claudia. *Woman-Centered Pregnancy and Birth.* Pittsburgh: Cleis Press.

Rozdilsky, Mary, and Barbara Banet. *What Now? A Handbook for New Parents.* New York: Scribner, 1975.

Scher, Jonathan, and Carol Dix. *Will My Baby Be Normal? How to Make Sure.* New York: Doubleday, 1983.

Stewart, David, and Lee Stewart. *Compulsory Hospitalization or Freedom of in Childbearing.* Marble Hill, Mo.: NAPSAC, 1978.

INDEX

Abdominal tightening exercise, 176; to reduce gas discomfort, 140–142, 145, 218
Activities, limitations on, following cesarean delivery, 165–167
Acupuncture, 107–108
Admitting routines, 98–103
Aesculapius, 197
Alcohol, use of, during pregnancy, 45, 46, 47
Allen, Ruth, xii, 207–209, 215, 216, 221
Aloe vera: to relieve itchiness of scar, 152; for stretch marks, 42
Alternative Birth Centers (ABCs), 2, 3, 28, 33, 180
Alveoli, 78
American Academy of Husband-Coached Childbirth, 248
American College of Home Obstetrics, 248
American College of Obstetrics and Gynecology (ACOG), 94, 225, 227–229

American Foundation for Maternal & Child Health, 248
American Journal of Obstetrics and Gynecology, 231
American Medical Association (AMA), 223, 224
American Society for Psychoprophylaxis in Obstetrics (ASPO), 249
Amniocentesis, 54, 80–83; to determine chromosomal abnormalities, 83–85; to determine fetal lung maturity, 85–88
Amniotic fluid, 80–82, 85
Amniotic sac, rupture of, 229
Anesthesia, 100, 102, 182; choice of, 108–109, 205; development of, 202; easier administration of, 109–111; types of, 103–108
Anesthesiologist, 103, 106
Anesthetist, 103
Anoxia, 13, 14, 18
Antisepsis, 202
Apgar, Dr. Virginia, 45, 125

Apgar score, 78, 124–125, 182
Apollo, 197
Aspiration pneumonia, 24
Association for Childbirth at
   Home, International, 249
Audio-visual aids, 221–222
Ausculation, 30

Backache, 43
Baths, limitation on, following
   cesarean delivery, 166–167
Bauhin, Caspar, 198
Bennet, Dr. Jesse, 201
"Bikini cut," 112, 153
Binder, 152
Bing technique, 53, 180
Biophysical profile, 90–91
Birth control, 167, 173–174;
   breast-feeding and, 189
Blood transfusions, 99, 117
Boland, Alice, 226
Boland, Donald and Dellann,
   226–227
Bonding, mother-infant, 106,
   109, 126, 137; importance of,
   178–186
Borg, Susan, *When Pregnancy
   Fails* (with J. Lasker), 220
Bradley method, 2, 238, 241, 248
Braxton Hicks contractions, 53,
   90, 94–95, 218
Breast-feeding, 2–3, 153, 168,
   184; in delivery room, 126,
   138–139, 205; and the Pill,
   167, 189; in recovery room,
   137, 138; significance of, to
   cesarean mothers and babies,
   187–192
Breath, shortness of, 41
Breathing techniques, *see*
   Relaxation breathing
   techniques
Breech presentation: as
   indication for cesarean

delivery, 10, 17–22; rotating,
   20–21
Brewer, Gail, *What Every
   Pregnant Woman Should
   Know,* 88–89
Brow presentation, 19

Caesar, Julius, 196–197
Cannula, 82
Car seats, baby, 160, 172
Catheter, 107, 137, 146; Foley,
   115
Catheterization, 115
Cervix, dilation of, 77
Cesarean Connection, 249
Cesarean delivery, previous, as
   indication for repeat cesarean,
   17, 32
Cesarean mother, image of
   typical, 35–37
Cesarean Prevention Movement,
   see CPM
"Cesarean shuffle," 146
Checklist, of choices to explore,
   203–206
Childbirth classes, 2, 53, 206;
   and cesarean revolution, 215–
   217; miscellaneous notes on,
   221–222; outline for, 217–
   221; prepared, 209–215
Childbirth Education Association
   (CEA), 130
Children: explaining cesarean
   delivery to, 57–58; visits to
   mother from, during
   postpartum hospital stay, 158,
   206
*China: The Other Half of the
   Sky,* 107
Chromosomal abnormalities,
   amniocentesis to determine,
   83–85
Cigarettes, smoking, during
   pregnancy, 45, 46, 47, 90

Circulation, poor, 40–41
Clarion, The, 226, 236
Clothing and equipment, baby, 172
Cohen, Nancy Wainer, *Silent Knife* (with L. J. Estner), 2, 234–235, 240, 243
Colic, 193
Colostrum, 139, 184, 192
Conception, estimated date of, 77
Constipation, 49, 146, 147, 193
Consumer Reports, 45
Contractions: Braxton Hicks, 53, 90, 94–95, 218; postpartum, 54
Contraction testing ("stress" testing), 89–90, 91
Controlled relaxation breathing, 54–55. *See also* Relaxation breathing techniques
Coronis, 197
Corticosteroids, 86
CPD (cephalopelvic disproportion), 79, 240; as indication for cesarean delivery, 17, 26–27
CPM (Cesarean Prevention Movement), 232, 233–234, 236, 249
Cragin, Dr., 230
Cramps, leg, 41
Craniotomy, 199, 201
Crying, baby's, 168, 169
C/SEC (Cesareans/Support, Education, and Concern), 216, 236, 249

Davis, Adele, 24
Dehiscence, 234
Delivery, 120–127; emotional stress after, 72–76; preparations for, 114–120; relaxation breathing techniques during, 53; room, father in, 128–132
Depression, postpartum, 73–76, 153–155
Diabetes, 28, 89; as indication for cesarean delivery, 10, 14, 15–16
Diana, Princess, of Great Britain, 3
Diarrhea, 193
Diet: after cesarean delivery, 146–148; during pregnancy, 47–51
Discomfort, coping with physical, during pregnancy, 39–45
Dissociative breathing and touch relaxation, 55–57. *See also* Relaxation breathing techniques
Dix, Carol, *Will My Baby Be Normal? How to Make Sure* (with J. Scher), 2, 84–85
Dizziness: after administration of anesthesia, 119–120; postpartum, 166
Doulas, 212
Dow, Dr. Nancy Edwards, 32, 33
Down's syndrome, 83
Driving, limitation on, following cesarean delivery, 165
Drugs, during pregnancy, 45–47, 90
Dystocia, as indication for cesarean delivery, 17, 22–26

Eclampsia, as indication for cesarean delivery, 14, 15
Ectopic pregnancy, 80
Edward, Prince, 196
Eileitheyria, 197
Elderly primigravidas, 33, 36. *See also* Older mothers
Electrocardiograph (EKG), 118

Elkins, Valmai, 141
Emergency cesarean, 9–11, 23
Enemas, 115
Epidural anesthesia, 100, 102,
    103–105, 108–109;
    administration of, 110–111;
    discussion of, 107
Episiotomy, 11
Equipment and clothing, baby,
    172
Erythromycin, 183
Estner, Lois J., *Silent Knife*
    (with N. W. Cohen), 2, 234–
    235, 240, 243
Estriol counts, 88
Exercise(s): abdominal
    tightening, to reduce gas
    discomfort, 140–142, 145,
    218; pelvic-floor (Kegals, 44–
    45, 221; postpartum, 175–
    176; during pregnancy, 43–45,
    51–53
External version, 20–21

Family-Centered Maternity Care
    (FCMC), 2, 3, 168, 180, 181,
    237; discussion of, 156–158
Fascia, 121
Father: in cesarean delivery
    room, 128–132, 205, 219; and
    decision to breast-feed, 191;
    and Family-Centered
    Maternity Care, 156, 157–158;
    infant care shared by, 170–
    171; significant role of, 2, 39,
    221; visiting hours for, 156,
    157, 206
Fear, *see* Stress, emotional
Felkin, 202
Fetal activity (movement)
    charting, 88, 90
Fetal distress, as indication for
    cesarean delivery, 17, 25,
    28–31

Fetal lung maturity,
    amniocentesis to determine,
    85–88
Fetal monitors, 28–31, 82
Fetopelvic disproportion, as
    indication for cesarean
    delivery, 17, 26–27
Fetoscope, 29, 30
Fonda, Jane, 53
Foods: limitation on spicy,
    following cesarean delivery,
    166; solid, starting babies on,
    192–194. *See also* Diet
Frustaci, Patricia and Samuel, 97
Frustration, 73
Fundal pressure, 121, 219
Fundus, height of, 77

Gas discomfort, 146, 147, 166;
    abdominal tightening exercise
    to reduce, 140–142, 145, 218
General anesthesia, 100, 103–
    105, 108–109; discussion of,
    106–107
Genetic counseling, 83–85
Genital herpes, active, as
    indication for cesarean
    delivery, 10, 14–15
German measles, 45
Gleicher, Dr. Norman, 223–225
Government Printing Office,
    U.S., 48
Grapefruit Syndrome, 4–6
Gynecology and Obstetrics, 198

Headaches, resulting from spinal
    anesthesia, 137
Health, Education and Welfare,
    U.S. Department of, 37
Heartburn, 40
Heart disease, maternal, as
    indication for cesarean
    delivery, 14, 16
Hemorrhage, as indication for
    cesarean delivery, 12

Hemorrhoids, 49
Henry VIII, King, 196
Herpes simplex, *see* Genital
herpes
Home birth, 3, 26, 240–245
Hormone testing, 91
Hospital: stay, postpartum, 143–
159; timing of admission to,
204. *See also* Admitting
routines
Hot flashes, 40; postpartum, 166
Human placental lactogen
(HPL), 91
Hyaline membrane disease, 78.
See also Respiratory Distress
Syndrome
Hypertension, 85, 89; and need
for cesarean delivery, 15
Hypnosis, 108
Hypotension, 104, 219
Hysterectomy, 199

Iatrogenic disease or problem,
17
ICEA (International Childbirth
Education Association), 232,
236
Illnesses, chronic, as indication
for cesarean delivery, 10
Incisions, 120–121; fears about
rupturing, 152, 174; healing
of, 152–153; itching of, 152;
sensations caused by, 146;
types of skin, 111–113
Incubator, 78
Indications, for cesarean
delivery, 7–12, 35–37;
mandatory, 12–14; probable,
14–16; reassurance about, 34–
35; relative or possible, 17–34
Induction, failed, as indication
for cesarean delivery, 17,
27–28
International Childbirth

Education Association, *see*
ICEA
Isolette, 78
IV (intravenous), 117, 135, 137,
146

"Johnny," 114
*Journal of the American Medical
Association (JAMA)*, 223, 224

Kaplan, Adam, 238, 241, 243,
244, 245
Kaplan, Bobby, 238, 239, 241,
243
Kaplan, Carey and Marc,
238–245
Kegals, *see* Pelvic-floor exercises
Kidney disease, *see* Renal
disease
Kitzinger, Sheila, 56, 247
Kitzinger technique, 53, 180
Korte, Diana, *A Good Birth, A
Safe Birth* (with R. Scaer),
232

Labor: alternative positions for,
in breech presentation, 21;
benefits of spontaneous, 95–
96; premature, 86; signs of,
93–95, 218; spontaneous, 22,
78–79. *See also* Dystocia
Labor attendants (LA's), 182
La Leche League, 187–188, 189,
236, 249
Lamaze method, 2, 53, 180, 238,
249
Lasker, Judith, *When Pregnancy
Fails* (with S. Borg), 220
Leboyer, Dr. Frederic, 183
Leboyer method, 2, 183
Lecithin, 85, 86
Leg cramps, 41
Lifting or carrying heavy objects,
limitation on, following
cesarean delivery, 165–166

Lochia, 151, 166. *See also*
    Vaginal discharge
Los Angeles Times, 237
Lubrication, lack of vaginal, 173

MacLaine, Shirley, 107
McTammany, Dr. J. Robert,
    129–131
Malpractice suits, 128, 129
Marijuana, use of, during
    pregnancy, 46, 47, 90
Mature mothers, *see* Older
    mothers
Meconium, 29
Medications: deciding in advance
    about, 25, 205; pain, after
    cesarean delivery, 148
Mendelsohn, Dr. Robert S., 212,
    225; *Confessions of a Medical
    Heretic,* 96; *Mal(e) Practice,*
    96, 211
Menstrual bleeding, breast-
    feeding and, 188–189
Mercurio, Scipone, 200–201
Milinaire, Catherine, *Birth,*
    45–46
Milk, arrival of mother's, 153
Mirror, to view cesarean birth,
    119, 205
Miscarriage, amniocentesis and,
    82, 84
Mongolism, 83
Monitresses, 212
Montague, Ashley, 156
Morning sickness, 49
Multiple births, as indication for
    cesarean delivery, 17, 31, 32
Myerscough, Dr. P. R., *Munro
    Kerr's Operative Obstetrics,*
    17–18
Mythological references, to
    cesarean delivery, 197

National Association of Parents
    & Professionals for Safe

Alternatives in Childbirth
    (NAPSAC), 249
National Foundation–March of
    Dimes, 45
National Institute of Child
    Health and Human
    Development Conference on
    Childbirth, 227
National Institutes of Health
    (NIH), 96, 223, 224, 225
Nausea, after administration of
    anesthesia, 119–120
Nembutal, 115, 219
Neonatologist, 97
Networking, 248
Newsweek, 225
Noble, Elizabeth, 53; *Essential
    Exercises for the Childbearing
    Years,* 141, 176
Nonstress testing, 88–89, 91
Normal (Natural) Birth Centers
    (NBCs), 2, 3, 28, 33
Norwood, Christopher, 33; *How
    to Avoid a Cesarean Section,*
    2, 240
NPO, 102
Nufer, Joseph, 199
Numa Pompilius, 197
Nursing, *see* Breast-feeding
Nutrition, *see* Diet

Odent, Dr. Michel, 226
Older (over thirty) mothers,
    special circumstances of, 17,
    32–34
Orgasm, 90; to release labor
    stimulant, 23
Oxygen, to combat nausea and
    dizziness, 120
Oxytocin, 23, 24
Oxytocin challenge testing, *see*
    Contraction testing

Pain(s): chest or rib, 40;
    medication for, after cesarean

delivery, 148; shoulder, resulting from surgery, 137
Palpating, of abdomen, 19
Pediatrician, visits with, 167–168
Pelvic contraction, maternal, as indication for cesarean delivery, 12, 13
Pelvic examinations, 53
Pelvic-floor exercises (Kegals), 44–45, 221
Pelvic insufficiency, as indication for cesarean delivery, 10
Pelvic rock, 23, 43–44
Pelvic tilt, 20
Peritoneum, 121
Pigmentation, extra, 41–42
Pitocin, 24, 27, 28, 31, 89; for contraction of uterus, 135
Pittsburgh, University of, 143
Placenta, 31, 45, 89, 91; delivery of, 126
Placenta abruptio, 120; as indication for cesarean delivery, 12–13
Placenta previa, 90; as indication for cesarean delivery, 12, 14, 16
Postmature baby, as indication for cesarean delivery, 17, 31
Postpartum contractions, 54
Postpartum discomfort, 54
Postpartum experience, *see* Trimester, fourth
Pregnancy, cesarean, 38–39; coping with physical discomfort during, 39–45; and delivery, explanation of, to children, 57–58; diet during, 47–51; drugs during, 45–47; exercise during, 43–45, 51–53; relaxation breathing techniques during, 53–57; role of father in, 39
Premature and low birth weight babies, as indication for cesarean delivery, 17, 32
Prepping, 99–100, 204–205
Principles and Practice of Obstetrics, 198
Prolapsed umbilical cord, *see* Umbilical cord

Quickening, 77

Ranney, Dr. Brooks, 20–21
Recovery room, time spent in, 133–140, 142, 219–220
Relaxation breathing techniques, 81, 90, 110, 145, 218, 221; discussion of, 53–57
Renal disease, 89; as indication for cesarean delivery, 14, 16
Respiratory Distress Syndrome (RDS), 22, 27, 78; and fetal lung maturity, 85, 86, 87–88
Rest, importance of, 151–152
Revolution, cesarean, 215–217
Rh factor incompatibility, as indication for cesarean delivery, 14, 16
Richmond, Dr. John L., 202
Ritodrine, 86, 95
Rooming-in, 2, 155–156, 185, 206
Roonhuyze, Hendrik von, 201
Rubin, Reeva, 143

Sanger, Max, 202
Sanitary pads, 150
Scaer, Roberta, *A Good Birth, A Safe Birth* (with D. Korte), 232
Scar: concerns about, 174; healing of, 152–153. *See also* Incisions
Scher, Dr. Jonathan, *Will My Baby Be Normal? How to Make Sure* (with C. Dix), 2, 84–85

Septuplets, birth of, 97–98
Sexuality: after delivery, 72, 167, 173–175; during pregnancy, 42–43
Seymour, Jane, 196
Silent Knife, see Cohen, Nancy Wainer; Estner, Lois J.
Silver nitrate, 183
Smoking, *see* Cigarettes
Snacks, nutritious, during pregnancy, 49–50
Snugli, 169, 172, 180–181
Sonogram, *see* Ultrasound
Sphingomyelin, 85
Spinal anesthesia, 100, 102, 103–105, 108–109; administration of, 110–111; discussion of, 107; headaches resulting from, 137
Stair climbing, limitation on, following cesarean delivery, 165
Stitches, 127. *See also* Incisions
Stress, emotional, 59–66; alleviating, with education and empathy, 66–72; after delivery, 72–76
Stress test, 54, 89–90
Stretch marks, 42
Support groups, 150, 171, 248–249
Supporting cesarean parents, 207–209
Surgical risks, from cesarean delivery, 230–231
Suturing, 126–127, 202

Tags, color-coded, on cribs of babies delivered by cesarean, 148–149
Tailor sitting, 43
Tay-Sachs disease, 84
Teenage mothers, *see* Young mothers
Teeth, cutting, 193

Terbutaline, 86
Tests, to determine fetal maturity and well-being, 32, 54, 77–79; amniocentesis, 80–88; biophysical profile, 90–91; contraction testing (stress testing), 89–90; deciding to submit to, 91–92; estriol counts, 88; fetal activity charting, 90; hormone testing, 91; nonstress testing, 88–89; ultrasound (sonogram), 79–80
Thalidomide scandal, 45
Thirst: after cesarean delivery, 147; of nursing mothers, 191–192
Time magazine, 129
Touching, advantages of early, 139, 168–169, 178–186
Toxemia, 28, 85, 89; defined, 15; and need for cesarean delivery, 14, 15
Tranquilizers, preoperative, 115–116
Transverse incision, 112–113, 121
Transverse lie, as indication for cesarean delivery, 12, 13–14
Trimester, fourth, 160–165, 167–173, 220–221; exercises during, 175–176; prohibitions during, 165–167; sex during, 173–175
Triplets, *see* Multiple births
Tubal ligation, 99, 127
Twins, *see* Multiple births

Ultrasound, 19, 20, 79–80, 91
Umbilical cord, 124, 167, 182; prolapsed, as indication for cesarean delivery, 12, 13
Urbanowski, Ferris, *Yoga for New Parents,* 53
USA Today, 237
Uterine dependability, 234–245

Uterus: contraction of, 135;
    prolapsed, 221; removal of,
    199, 202

Vaginal birth after cesarean, *see*
    VBAC
Vaginal delivery, differences
    between cesarean section and,
    1, 35
Vaginal discharge, postpartum,
    134, 145, 151, 166
Vaginal infection, 40
Valium, 115, 219
VBAC (vaginal birth after
    cesarean), xiii, 27, 66, 206,
    223–232; advantages of, 2;
    classes, 233–234; information
    about, 68, 70, 71; and uterine
    dependability, 234–245
Vegetarian mothers-to-be, 49
Vena cava, 30, 41, 55, 118
Vernix, 124
Vertex presentation, 19, 20
Vertical midline (classical)
    abdominal incision, 112–113,
    153
Visiting hours, 156, 157, 206

Vital signs, 99, 134
Vitamins and minerals: during
    pregnancy, 47–48, 51;
    following surgery, 147–148
Vomiting, after administration
    of anesthesia, 119

Walking, as exercise during
    pregnancy, 52
Wall Street Journal, 237
Williams Obstetrics, 197
Willughby, Percival, "The
    Country Midwife's Opusculum
    on Vade Mecum," 200
"Window," 234

X-rays, 79

Yoga, 56; during pregnancy, 53
Young (under twenty) mothers,
    special circumstances of, 17,
    32–34

Zorn, Esther Booth, 233,
    236–237
Zorn, Maximillian, 236, 237